JimsHealthAndMuscle.com

Chair workouts for every fitness level

Chair exercise for strength, movement & balance. Quick seated workouts with fitness results in mind.

James Atkinson

ISBN: 978-0-9932791-9-5

JBA Publishing

Copyright © 2024

JimsHealthAndMuscle.com

Contents

Why chair workouts?..1

Health Check...3

Getting started with chair workouts 4

Type of chair to use..11

Chair yoga 14

Adding resistance..22

Workload and fitness goals 26

Exercise routine planning..30

Weight loss & muscle toning routine 32

Exercise for Longevity and function 52

Exercise for strength and muscle gain 68

Your personalised routine 94

Progression 99

More exercises...101

Back 102

Legs...108

Arms 116

Shoulders 126

Abdominals 134

Yoga poses...142

Would you like to help me out? 156

Something else you may be interested in? 157

Also by James Atkinson 158

Blank Program Cards 162

Why chair workouts?

Mainstream gyms, personal trainers and even home gyms can be excellent for fitness goals and progression. Not everyone, however, has access to these facilities or indeed the ability to perform comfortably in these environments. This doesn't mean that the chance to engage in exercise and fitness has to be denied.

Chair workouts are an excellent exercise solution for:

- Senior fitness
- Rehabilitation
- People who have issues with standing
- People with limited movement
- Many wheelchair users

Despite the list above, anyone can use chair exercise for development of:

- Circulation
- Flexibility
- Strength
- Cardio
- Functional movements
- Balance

Although we are seated during a chair workout routine, we can still engage and indeed challenge every muscle group, including the lower body. For trainers with limited lower body function, or trainers that have problems with balance, having the knowledge of lower body muscle engagement while seated gives a unique opportunity to perform exercises in this area.

Chair workouts may not be optimum for goals such as strong man competitions, bodybuilding shows or track and field events, but it is not to say that these types of fitness goals are completely out of the question, as we will explore later in the guide.

Chair exercise is, however, excellent for the most fundamental and, in my opinion, the most important form of fitness. This is functional strength and mobility.

With the development of good functional strength and mobility, we will find everyday tasks easier. Also by moving our bodies through ranges of movement that they were designed to move through will challenge our joints and muscles responsible for these movements to keep them active.

For more clarity on functional strength and mobility, a common problem area for many people is shoulder muscle weakness. This is because most everyday activities don't call for overhead reaches or lifts. This can cause weakness in the deltoids and shoulder girdle. Another common issue is that many people will neglect to use certain muscle groups when performing everyday activities. This can be for many reasons, including pain in certain planes of movement, but it can also be because of weaknesses in certain muscle groups. An example of this is the simple act of sitting on a chair. To sit on a chair, we should use several muscle groups, including quads (upper legs), core (abdominals and lower back), and glutes. But rather than engage these muscles, it's much easier to take our body weight by leaning on the chair, turning around and letting gravity take its course.

Cardio exercise is also possible with chair workouts. The idea behind cardio fitness is to challenge the heart and lungs through sustained movement. By using functional movements from a seated position dynamically, we can put our bodies in a state of cardiovascular development. This basically uses the single chair exercise movements in a different cadence, merging function with cardio. The guide includes a more thorough explanation of this later.

In this guide, we will cover these concepts in more detail and by the end of the book; you will have the knowledge and be well equipped to perform effective chair workouts with the following fitness goals in mind:

- Weight loss and muscle toning
- Longevity and function
- Strength and muscle gain

Let's get started!

Health Check

Before you embark on any fitness routine, please consult your doctor or physiotherapist. If you have any health conditions, always check if the type of exercise and exercise choices you intend to involve yourself with.

1.   Do not exercise if you are unwell.

2.   Stop if you feel pain, and if the pain does not subside, consult your doctor or physiotherapist.

3.   Do not exercise if you have taken alcohol or had a large meal in the last few hours.

4.   If you are taking medication, please check with your doctor to make sure it is okay for you to exercise.

5.   If in doubt at all, please check with your doctor or physiotherapist first – you may even want to take this routine and go through it with them. It may be helpful to ask for a blood pressure, cholesterol and weight check. You can then have these taken again in a few months to see the benefit.

Getting started with chair workouts

There is a fair amount of material in this guide and points made that can easily be overlooked or bypassed in order to follow an exercise routine. Although I try my best to explain everything in layman's terms with a logical, structured approach, for the total beginner, it may still be slightly overwhelming.

With that said, if you only read one section, or take a single piece of information away from this chair workouts guide, this should be it.

As a long-term health and fitness practitioner with formal qualifications and a career backing this up, I have always given priority to range of motion and posture in my own training and that of my clients. Whether the fitness goal is fat loss, endurance running or indeed bodybuilding, whatever the goal, this should be the foundation. Chair workouts are no different. In fact, I would go as far as saying that the "default position" (this will be covered in this section) will be an isometric exercise in itself for some trainers.

Let's talk about this "default position". The first thing that we should do is prepare our mind-set. This may sound like a formality, or something that can be overlooked. But practicing this is important, and we should do it before and during every exercise session for optimal results. Even though chair workouts are considered low intensity, low impact, and gentle workouts, we should still go into each session with a workout mentality.

With chair workouts, this starts with the mind-set switching to "workout mode". This mode turns on when we are setting up our workout chair. It stays on throughout the entire training session and turns off only after the last exercise is complete and we are putting our chair away.

Workout mode

"Workout mode" is a term I use, but other trainers and instructors probably have their own take on it. To explain this in a chair exercise capacity, here is a rundown of how to approach each exercise session:

Prepare your equipment – Before every workout, you should make sure you have everything in place. You should:

- Have your routine card or plan (we will create these later)
- Have your equipment, including your chair and any other pieces of workout kit needed for your workout. There may be some exercises that you choose to use extra resistance, such as resistance bands or small weights.
- Have an allotted time frame when you won't be disturbed. This is your time and no one else's
- Always maintain or revert back to the default posture throughout the session. When we are sitting on the chair in these workouts, this will ensure we are still in "workout mode" and are ready for the next exercise

Default position

It's been mentioned a lot already, and it will be referred to throughout the guide, and it is going to be the "exercise" that we will spend most of our time performing. Yes, I called this an exercise, as I believe it is just that. Here is a rundown of the all-important "default position".

Prepare to sit

Believe it or not, we start before we have even sat on the chair. Position your chair so you have room for all exercises. You should be able to reach out to your sides, above your head and have no obstructions for your legs to stretch out. Turn so the chair is behind you in a position you would normally be in if you were to sit on it. Your feet should be about hip width apart.

Your shoulders should be pulled back and down to open up your chest and your head should be facing forward.

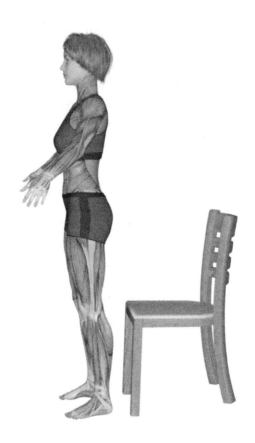

Take a seat

Once in this position, it's time to sit down. As you exhale and engage your abdominals, slowly bend at the knees and hinge at the hips, keeping your back flat. You can choose to raise your arms to the front for counter balance if you wish. You should feel your quads engage. This is technically part of the squat exercise that can be used for repetition for upper leg strength within your workouts. This is included in section 2 as an exercise choice.

Lowering to the seated position should be a slow and controlled movement. The aim is to maintain control until you are sitting on the chair. If you can pause and hold at any point of this movement, you have mastered it!

Between reps and different exercise movements, we may not need to repeat this step, but we should be aware of it throughout the workout as some exercises may call for movement away from the chair to set up extra equipment such as resistance bands or dumbbells.

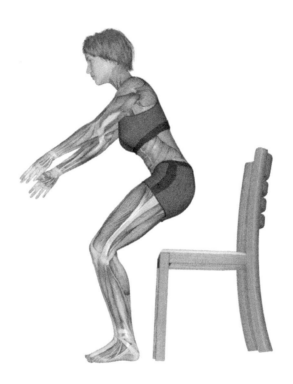

In position, ready!

Now that we are sitting down, before we start any exercise, we should reassess our position and adjust if needed.

- Feet should be flat on the floor, ankles directly below our knees

- Back should be flat and not rounded. We sit tall and engage our abdominals.
- Shoulders should be pulled back and down
- Head should be facing forward
- Our main body weight should be concentrated through our glutes to the seat of the chair
- Arm position will vary depending on the exercise, but resting by our sides is a good default

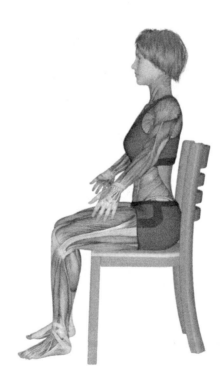

You can practise this procedure every time you sit on a chair during everyday life. The act of sitting on a chair in this way engages a range of big muscle groups, including stabiliser muscles that aid with balance.

Core engagement

In all of my previous exercise guides and my home workout video course, I have repeatedly used a phrase, probably to the point it is worn out:

"Keep your abs tight"

I feel that this is important during most aspects of exercise. I also believe I've taken for granted that people know what this means, so here is a more in-depth explanation.

Tightening your abdominal muscles isn't simply "crunching your stomach muscles". This act is ok for some as the deeper core will engage by doing this, but for total beginners or people who have a weak core, there is a better way to activate this correctly.

Once we are sitting in the start position, we take a deep breath in. We then exhale slowly. Just as we hit the point that our lungs are empty, we try to exhale further. At this point, we should feel our stomach flatten.

This "flattening of the stomach" is the engagement we are looking for. Once we feel this, we can use the movement to visualise our belly button being drawn inwards towards our spine. We can now hold this engagement through our abdominals and carry on breathing normally.

Now we are "keeping our abs tight!"

Like the other stages of the default position, we can practise this breathing technique and abs engagement as its own exercise. The more we do this, the more natural it will feel.

To sum this up:

- Make sure you are prepared before each workout, mentally and physically
- The default position is important. We will be spending most of our workout session in this position
- Always be aware of your posture before starting any exercise and reset if necessary

- Always maintain the default position when resting between exercises. This will keep us in "workout mode" whilst also engaging important muscle groups
- Sitting on a chair can be an exercise on its own, so it's a transferable skill for everyday life
- It will be extremely beneficial to practise each stage of the default position, especially if there is an aspect of the process that's particularly challenging for you

Type of chair to use

It is possible to use any chair for chair exercise, but there are optimal choices and the first thing to consider is safety. Chairs with wheels such as office chairs are not ideal, especially if we are training with resistance bands or dumbbells, as we need a solid foundation. Disability wheelchairs are an option, as most have a break to secure the chair in place. If you are using such a chair, always make sure to fully apply the brake before you start the workout. Sofas, armchairs and other chairs with heavy cushioning are not ideal as they tend to be restrictive and don't offer the support that we need during many exercises.

The best type of chair for chair exercise should:

- Be sturdy in construction
- Have none slip feet
- Have a flat seat
- Not have arm rests
- Have an upright, solid back rest

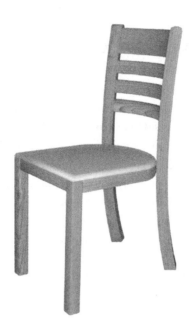

Solid dining room style chairs are a great choice. All the illustrations in this guide depict this type of chair. If you are a wheelchair user but have access to this type of chair and can use it comfortably, without issue, this would be a better option.

Although the backrest is not used in most exercises, it's still advisable to have one. For the total beginner, this acts as a safety barrier and offers reassurance on certain exercises that call for an adjusted position that angles the upper body backwards.

If you do not have access to a chair with a backrest, and wish to train with bodyweight exercises, placing a backless chair that meets the other criteria against a wall is a good option. The more advanced we become with chair workouts; the less need there will be for a backrest.

Although this is not accessible for the majority of us without a gym membership, it's worth mentioning another great option for seated workouts is a standard gym bench. A good workout bench is an excellent choice, as it offers great stability with a narrow seat and minimal obstructions.

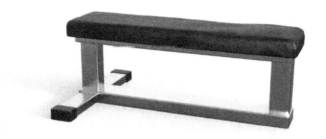

For advanced trainers, exercise balls are often used for full seated workouts. This type of seat offers a whole new dimension to a training session. Sitting on an exercise ball requires an engagement of many stabiliser muscles. Maintaining good form during each exercise becomes all the more challenging as we are always working against the unstable platform. Mobility, balance and general fitness goals are probably the most appropriate for exercise ball workouts. I would not, however, advise using an exercise ball as a seat for strength training or muscle gain goals, as these goals require exercise choices and methods that do not work well with this setup.

Performing seated workouts on an exercise ball is an excellent upgrade for those wishing to take things to the next level of their mobility and stability fitness goals. Moving directly from a solid chair or workout bench to an exercise ball might be too big a step for some, so there are options to make this transition a bit smoother. It is possible to acquire a support or base specifically designed for exercise balls that transforms them into a more stable seat. This may be worth more investigation if you wish to go down this route.

The most important thing when choosing a chair to workout with is that it is sturdy, has a flat seat and is unlikely to slip on the floor.

Chair yoga

A quick preface to any serious yogis and yoginis that may stumble upon this text: I appreciate the art of yoga and what it stands for, so there is no intention of diminishing this practice. For the purpose of this guide, I intend to simply highlight the benefits of the physical part of yoga by stripping it back to muscle function and body mechanics often associated with yoga. ☺

Yoga and chair yoga is an excellent activity for the development of balance, functional strength, range of movement and mind muscle connection. But what differentiates yoga from other exercise forms, and what are the similarities? In this short section, we answer this question while breaking down a popular form of yoga and suggesting options to incorporate chair yoga into a workout routine.

These days, in the mainstream health, fitness and exercise space, yoga is widely considered, simply as a form of exercise. It's probably hard to define yoga without having considerable experience in its ways, and it would probably take more than a sentence to do it, but here is my attempt: The true reason to perform yoga sessions is rooted in spirituality and the search for enlightenment. So it's all about mind, body, spirit and the connection to all things.

The draw to yoga, and indeed chair yoga for most people, is the fact that this exercise technique works the body in a low impact, functional way using little or no exercise equipment. It is extremely accessible, as the only tools that are needed are our own bodies.

If you bought this guide, you are obviously interested in seated exercise or chair workouts, but chair yoga might be something that you may have considered or you would like to investigate more. So in this section I will explain how yoga poses when stripping them back to the physical benefits are functional movements to develop mobility, balance and a degree of muscle strength for function.

There are many "chair yoga" books, video courses and other guides on the market these days, and I know that most of these are fundamentally "chair workout books" using static poses taken from yoga. There is nothing wrong with this way of working the body; in fact, the physical benefits that come from performing yoga poses are excellent for almost everybody. There are some yoga poses for you to incorporate into your workouts detailed in section 2.

Although yoga can be used to move joints and develop mobility by performing controlled, repetitive range of motion movements (which is an excellent activity for everyone), I would like to focus on the "static hold" component that is associated with yoga as moving into these positions addresses mobility too.

I would like to give a rundown of the difference between repetitive exercises (the main focus of this guide) and yoga poses in this chapter. It may be that you would prefer to use static movements, or these may be a better fit for you for certain muscle groups. An understanding of static poses will enable you to modify them and other exercises if you have an issue with a certain aspect of the pose or exercise.

Generally, yoga poses will challenge several muscle groups and joint movements at the same time. I would like to invite you to follow the breakdown of a classic chair yoga pose to highlight that this is simply a functional movement that can be modified.

This yoga pose is a variation known as "Warrior". It has been adapted for chair workouts:

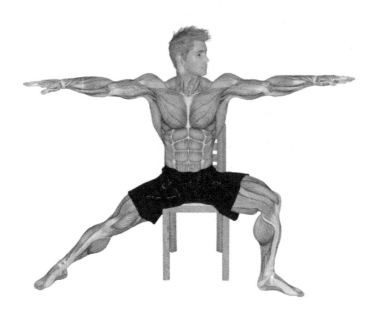

This single pose challenges many muscle groups and functions, including:

- Neck/ trap muscles and mobility
- Shoulder muscles and shoulder mobility
- Biceps mobility
- Chest opening
- Core stability
- Glutes and hip rotation
- Inner leg flexibility
- Outer leg flexibility
- Hamstring flexibility
- Calf flexibility
- Ankle mobility

As you can see, this exercise challenges a lot of areas of the body at once and there's much to think about when performing these types of holds. Yes, yoga poses are an excellent form of functional development, but they can be a bit overwhelming for the beginner. Having to concentrate when training a single muscle group can be challenging, as, even then, there are several things that you have to consider throughout the movement.

With this said, the nature of a yoga is connectivity and oneness, so concentrating on multiple muscle groups, connecting to each other, while working at the same time is a great definition of the art, that challenges the mind as well as the body.

As we are stripping back yoga to its physical component in this guide, we can, however, use parts of these yoga poses to cut down on the overwhelm. An example of this could be to perform the part of the exercise that targets the upper body only:

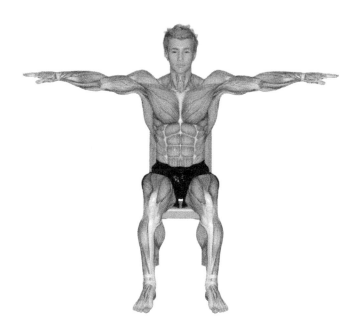

By doing a "partial warrior" pose, from our default position, we are simply raising our arms so they are parallel to the floor, palms facing down. This allows us to focus on this area more intently. We still have to maintain our posture and core engagement, but it is far more forgiving.

The act of raising our arms into this position can be used in a repetitive method, too. This engages the shoulder muscles and is known as a lateral raise. From this position, we can also make rotational movements with our shoulder joint to develop mobility in this area.

As you can see, there is a fine line between a yoga pose and a static hold where muscle function and mobility are concerned.

Static holds vs. dynamic movements

Static holds - A static hold is also known as an isometric exercise. We put our bodies into a position and hold for varying amounts of time. We can do this while working against gravity or adding an additional resistance such as a dumbbell or pushing against a solid object like a wall or door frame. The effect on the muscle groups being worked this way strengthens them in the position that they are in while the hold is maintained. We can have static holds at any point of a muscle's range of motion.

Here is an example of a static hold at two different positions for the bicep muscle:

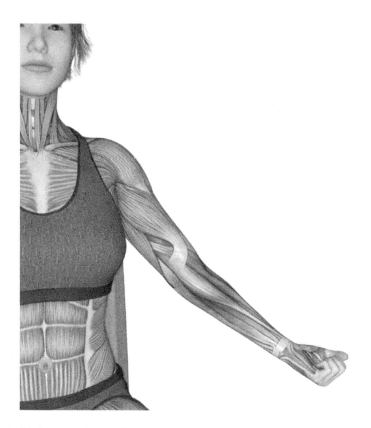

If we hold this position and engage our bicep we are strengthening the muscle in its elongated state.

We can do the same thing, but with our muscle in its contracted state:

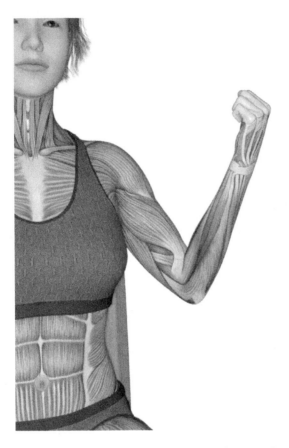

This works for every muscle group in the body, including stabiliser muscles and core.

Static holds and isometric exercise are often prescribed by physiotherapists to clients who are recovering from injury. This is because static holds often include tendon conditioning as well.

Dynamic movements- Dynamic exercises are exercises that move a muscle group through a full range of motion, usually working against gravity with bodyweight or with additional resistance added such as barbells, dumbbells or resistance bands.

Sticking with the example of the bicep, to challenge this muscle using a dynamic or isotonic exercise would be to perform a bicep curl. If we elongated our bicep by straightening our arm, held a dumbbell in our hand, engaged our bicep before contracting (bending at the elbow), then slowly returned to the start position, we would have performed a single rep of a bicep curl.

As we worked the muscle through its full range of motion, we would be strengthening it at every point of the movement.

So which is better, isometric exercise or isotonic exercise? The answer is neither. They both have great benefits. I would advise that you consider merging both forms into your workout plan. There are examples of full body routines set out later on in the guide that do this. Using both methods will help you to address problem areas that you may have and it will give you a more rounded fitness results.

I believe that understanding the difference between these two exercise methods is a valuable endeavour that can add variety to training sessions. Practicing dynamic movements will have a positive effect on the ability to perform static holds or yoga poses and vice versa.

Practicing yoga poses will also give us a better ability to feel a "mind muscle" connection when performing dynamic movements.

In summary, yoga and indeed chair yoga is an excellent activity for the development of mobility, functional muscle strength and mind muscle connection. There are many different styles of yoga, but static poses are commonly used and easily accessible. We can use full body yoga poses in our workouts, but these can also be broken down into partial movements. Practicing yoga poses will challenge our range of movement and give us a better understanding of body mechanics by moving the body through its full range.

Adding resistance

Exercising without equipment is very viable and can be a lifelong training method, but there is a certain point that we will reach where extra resistance or intensity is needed for further development. Adding resistance to an exercise will increase the workload to enable us to develop a muscle group further.

Learning an exercise movement will give us the range of motion and basic functional strength. This is the first step for everyone, whether this is someone who is in rehabilitation, a total beginner to fitness and exercise, or even a budding power lifter.

Once we have developed good exercise form and are comfortable with the movement, we can start to add extra resistance over time. Of course, this is entirely optional. We do not have to add resistance at all, but it's an efficient way of increasing strength and functional ability while working at our originally planned rep and set range.

This chair workout exercise guide focuses on exercises that target specific muscle groups, working them through repetition. These movements can be performed without resistance, but the exercise choices listed in section 2 have been selected so resistance can be added easily.

When adding resistance to an exercise, we are simply working against gravity with an additional force, or creating a resistance through a plane of movement to challenge the muscle where gravity is not a factor. There are many ways to add the "additional force". We could use everyday items such as food tins, bottles of water, bags of sand, or appropriate exercise equipment like hand weights, dumbbells, or resistance bands. For this type of exercise, I would suggest resistance bands as these are inexpensive, easy to store and have a huge versatility scope. A good set of resistance bands will last a long time and give us the potential for significant fitness progression.

Let's look at some examples of the same exercise performed with different methods of resistance:

Raising the arms to the sides from the default position engages the shoulder muscles. This is known as a "lateral raise". This movement is used in the variation of the warrior yoga pose that was detailed in the previous chapter, so the same muscle groups are being used. Without additional resistance, the exercise looks like this:

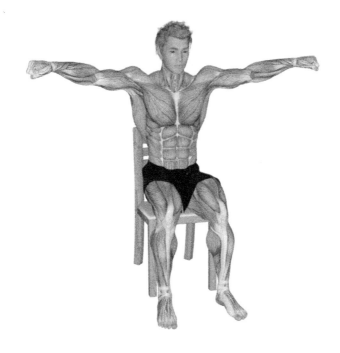

If we are able to hold this position for a set time frame or complete our target sets and reps range comfortably, we may want to challenge ourselves further to increase strength and stamina in the shoulder muscles. This is where we could explore additional resistance.

If we had access to free weights, we could do exactly the same movement but with the added resistance of dumbbells. Even the lightest set of dumbbells would give us an extra challenge if we were working within the same workload, i.e. the same amount of sets and reps or time frame.

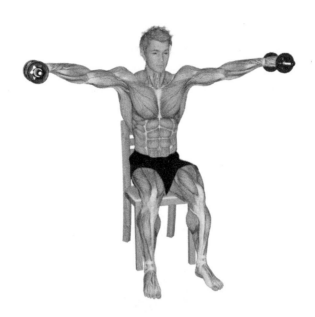

This is the same lateral raise exercise, but performed with dumbbells. Body position and range of movement are exactly the same, but with the added resistance.

The same movement can be performed with exercise bands. It looks like this:

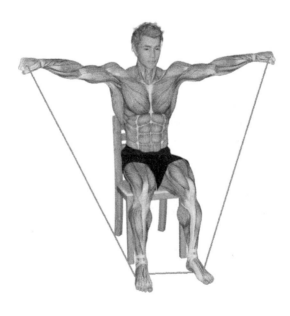

The difference here is that we would anchor the exercise bands with our feet. To do this, we always make sure the resistance band has equal lengths on either side of our feet and we make sure that the band isn't slack at our starting position. With some exercises, it might be necessary to grip the band nearer the anchor point rather than using any hand stirrups to achieve resistance from the start position.

Exercise bands are available in many thicknesses. Most sets are colour coordinated for quick identification.

When selecting a set of dumbbells, exercise bands or other forms of resistance, it's important that we don't sacrifice exercise form for a higher resistance level. I believe that exercise form should be the priority in any routine.

Developing a good range of movement and functional strength may be the ultimate goal for some. This is a good goal for everyone, but if you would like to challenge yourself past this goal, I would suggest using resistance bands as the next step. As mentioned before, these are excellent pieces of kit that can be used for every body part, and as they are widely available and fairly inexpensive, they are very accessible for everyone. It's for this reason that I have added variations of chair exercises using bands to section 2 in this guide.

If you feel that you are progressing well with a certain exercise, or you are stronger in certain areas than others, you may want to add a resistance band exercise to challenge that muscle group further. I am a big advocate of progression with workouts and adding resistance is a sure-fire way to achieve this.

Workload and fitness goals

Set out in this guide are several workout routines. Each routine is designed to promote a certain fitness result, or "fitness effect". If we train consistently with the same workload, over time we will see the benefits take form on our bodies. The way we train will determine what these benefits will be, so the workload needs to align with the fitness goals we have.

For clarity, I have always used the analogy of an ultra-marathon training routine and a competing bodybuilders' training routine. These fitness goals are at opposite ends of the fitness scale and they represent extreme goals. One is focused on cardio and endurance and the other is focused on intense resistance training. A long-distance runner's training routine will be drastically different from that of a competing bodybuilder and vice versa.

The point is that if a trainer wanted to compete in a bodybuilding show, and he trained for ultra-marathons using long cardio training sessions and endurance as his training method, he would not stand a chance against the other bodybuilders in his competition who have aligned their training with their goals, but he would beat the entire line up at by a long shot in a long distance running race. This works both ways.

We are probably not looking to be bodybuilders or long-distance runners, but the extremes of this example offer a clearer picture of the importance of aligning workload with our fitness goals.

I have seen this misalignment creep into many trainers' workout routines in a more subtle way than the above example. If we are simply looking to become more mobile, have better balance and feel fitter, as long as we move our bodies and joints through their range of motion regularly, and we are more active than we were, we will be on the right track. But if our goals are more specific and we don't align our training to match them, the big problem is that we won't see the results we want and in my experience, this causes disappointment or frustration which can lead to an abandonment of the workout routine.

To take the guesswork out of this for you, and to ensure that you are training for your goal, I have designed several routines that align with common fitness goals.

26

- Weight loss and muscle toning (full-body workout – Timed sets and circuit)
- Exercise for longevity and function (Full body - functional movements and Yoga)
- Strength and muscle gain (Pre exhaust sets with resistance bands)
- Rehabilitation to address common injury areas like lower back, shoulders/ bicep and also manage knee and neck pain

Here's a simple breakdown of each of these goals and what we should do in our workouts to align the exercise with the goal and explain why we are doing what we are doing in layman's terms

Exercise for weight loss and muscle toning

To achieve a weight loss and muscle toning fitness goal, we should first increase our heart rate for a sustained period. This is can be achieved by performing constant movement. An elevated heart rate uses energy, and using energy burns body fat if our diet is on point. Challenging our bodies by moving them through their various ranges of motion activates our muscles, which can tone and strengthen muscle. We can add extra resistance, such as exercise bands or dumbbells, for an extra challenge and to further progression. A positive side effect of resistance training is that the more lean muscle we have, the more energy our bodies will use during daily activities. This means there is an additional fat loss benefits.

The workload and method for this goal:

- Use timed exercises – 30 seconds to 1 minute per exercise
- Train full body in each workout
- 30 – 45 minute workouts (Continuous or circuit)
- Add resistance to where possible

Exercise for Longevity and function

Function and longevity is something we should all consider. If we don't challenge our muscle groups and the range of movement regularly, we run the risk of muscle atrophy and development of mobility problems. A regular exercise routine based on moving our bodies in the way they were designed to will promote mobility while developing and maintaining muscle strength.

Static holds and stretching exercises are going to be the focus of this type of exercise routine, although some sets and reps can be added for certain exercises.

The workload and method for this goal:

- Use timed exercises – 30 seconds to 1 minute per exercise
- Train partial or full body in each workout
- Workout length is subject to the individual
- Resistance can be added to some movements, but this is not essential

Exercise for strength and muscle gain

When the goal is strength and muscle gain, we should challenge the muscle group in question with resistance. This resistance could be bodyweight or equipment, such as free weights or bands. The key to developing muscle strength and size is in the workload and intensity. Generally, for each exercise, we should work in sets of 3-4 and repetitions of 12-15 while using a resistance that puts us close to failure on our last few reps. Failure being the point where we can't complete a rep without using full range of movement or we can't maintain our exercise form.

The workload and method for this goal:

- Use "sets and reps" training method
- Train partial or full body workouts
- Workout length is subject to the individual
- Additional resistance should be used to overload the muscle

Exercise for rehabilitation

The vast majority of people will suffer from injuries, muscle pain and stiffness, or arthritis in their lives. Back, shoulder, neck and knees are among the most common areas that need rehabilitation attention. When rehabbing a body part, the exercise needs to be gentle, progressive, and centred around movement and light resistance.

The workload and method for this goal:

** These are points for general guidance. Rehabilitation is specific to the individual. A trip to see a physiotherapist is advisable and can be extremely valuable if your goals are rehabilitation.

- Use sets, reps and timed static holds
- Train problem areas and synergist muscle groups
- Workout length dictated by the volume of training
- Additional resistance can be used, subject to the exercise. Resistance bands are widely used in rehabilitation routines

Following the guidelines for these goals is a great start. This can be followed directly, but it is certainly not "one size fits all" advice. For a better fit, you may wish to simply pick exercises from each of the workouts listed in the next chapter and add some extra exercise from the descriptions towards the end of the book to your own workout.

If an exercise choice looks interesting to you, or a method of working out appeals to you more than others, give it a go! Whatever your goal or training method is going to be, I would always advise that you fill in an exercise card as part of your plan. Do not underestimate the importance of this planning and prep activity.

Exercise routine planning

In this chapter, we'll look at workout routines that will align with the most common fitness goals mentioned in the previous section. You can follow along directly or alter the exercises within the workouts if you wish.

I have always been an advocate of creating a plan before starting any fitness venture, even if this is for the rehabilitation of a single muscle group or injury with few exercises. I have even created workout cards for people who are not that serious about getting results, as I know it will give them a boost in motivation.

The reason for this type of planning is that fitness results, whether they are muscle building, strengthening or cardio based goals, only ever come from structure and consistency. So if we have a plan in place, we simply have to execute it.

To help with this planning, I have designed simple routine cards that feature in all of my workout guides. Granted, these are slightly modified for this guide and for each training type, but the fundamentals are the same.

Filling out or simply copying one of the routine cards in this book will not only show us the path to our goals, but will also give us a vital tool to use in the creation of structure, consistency, accountability and motivation.

These workout routine cards are filled out with the following information:

- **Our fitness goals.** To keep this in our minds and remind us why we are doing what we are doing. I recommend looking into this a bit deeper for trainers with serious weight loss and diet goals, as it can be extremely powerful.

- **The routine number we are on.** This is helpful to keep track of over a long period, or for use in a split training routines. Over several months or even years of consistent training, we are more than likely going to upgrade our routine cards as we become fitter or our goals change. It's very useful to be able to look back on older routine cards to see how we have progressed or pick up on something we are missing.

- **Muscle group trained**. Understanding the benefits of an exercise on the body will make us more capable and knowledgeable of exercise in general. By listing the muscle groups worked on a routine card, we can choose these entries based on what we need to work on and to also ensure we are not neglecting an area. This is especially useful when working with full body routines.

- **Exercise**. Listing exercises is useful for quick reference during a training session so we don't forget what exercise comes next or indeed, miss an exercise altogether in our workouts. It's also useful to be able to list exercises in the order we would like to perform them. The order of exercise can make a big difference to the intensity of a workout, especially for exercise methods, such as circuit training.

- **Sets / reps / time**. Working within a "set & rep" range can be a general rule for an entire workout, or the range can be adjusted for specific exercises. This is useful to have on our routine cards, not only for quick reference during a workout but for monitoring progress. Training exercises with a sets and reps method can be switched for training within a time frame. This will depend on the fitness goal.

- **Training schedule**. This is really important for those who want to achieve optimum results. On this card design, we can mark our planned training days for up to six weeks ahead of time. Doing this will enable us to plan our training sessions every week and give us a measure of accountability.

I have always believed that planning in this way, having a physical copy of a routine (not something on a digital device) and reassessing regularly is very valuable as it plays a huge part in the outcome of a fitness venture. It should never be overlooked. I am more than happy to help anyone reading this book with the planning process and even the creation of a routine, so if something doesn't make sense, and you would like more guidance, please feel free to contact me.

Weight loss & muscle toning routine

"Weight loss and muscle tone" is probably the most common of fitness goals. In fact, muscle tone and sensible body fat percentage, in my opinion should be a goal taught to everyone from an early age as a matter of necessity. This goes far beyond body image and the visual aesthetics that come from the goal. The general health benefits and quality of life that are associated with this type of body composition are countless. So it is understandable why this is a common fitness aim.

Based on the guidelines outlined in the "workload & fitness goals" chapter, to achieve this result, we should:

- Use timed exercises
- Train full body in each workout
- Perform continuous movements

The routine that follows is designed with fat loss and muscle toning in mind. We use constant movement switching immediately from one exercise to the next without a break until we have completed all exercises. In this example, the full circuit should last about four minutes. We then have a two-minute break and repeat. The example shows that we perform this routine "4" times. However, depending on your fitness level, you may wish to adjust this. Keep in mind that the more sets we perform per workout, the more energy we will expend, making it more optimal for this particular fitness goal.

Our current fitness level is also an important consideration. It may be that we are over exerted after a single circuit and we need to stop. This is no problem and actually an excellent reason for having a workout card like this. We can always aim to improve. If we are consistent and keep the training pushing, we will see that this changes within a few weeks.

This is what the routine looks like:

WEIGHT LOSS & MUSCLE TONING			

ROUTINE #		

MUSCLE GROUP	EXERCISE	TIME	SETS
LEGS, CORE	ALTERNATE TOE TAP	30	
CHEST, LEGS, CORE	TOE TAP & FLYS	30	
LEGS, SHOULDERS	SEATED JACKS	30	
BICEPS, LEGS	TOE TAP, BICEP CURL	30	**4**
SHOULDERS, LEGS	TOE TAP, LATERAL RAISE	30	
BACK	REACH & PULL	30	
ABS	ALTERNATE ELBOW TO KNEE	30	
ABS	DOUBLE KNEE TO CHEST	30	
	2 MINUTE REST AND RESTART		

WEEKS	MON	TUE	WED	THURS	FRI	SAT	SUN
1	*			*			
2	*			*			
3	*		*		*		
4	*		*		*		
5	*		*		*	*	
6	*		*		*	*	

33

How it works – This is a circuit style workout. Before we start the session, we should have a stopwatch style timer that counts down in a continuous 30 second pattern. We start the first exercise and continue until the timer reaches zero, then immediately start the next exercise. Carry on like this until we reach the end of the exercise list. We then have a two-minute break and repeat until we have completed the number of sets we planned. The more familiar we are with the exercise choices, the better this style of workout will flow. It can be a bit clunky at first, but this is all part of the progression.

The training schedule on this example workout is set over six weeks. As you can see by the "*" marked in the boxes, this is upgraded to add extra session on a two-week basis. You could use this directly, but you may find that you can progress quicker, so feel free to adjust accordingly.

Tempo – As the fitness goal is "lose weight and tone muscle", the tempo of this workout is important if it is to align with the goal. The faster you make the movements, the more reps you will fit into each exercise, but with any exercise movement, we should always aim for a full range of movement and ensure that we are always in control by engaging the appropriate muscle group. So the best way to gauge tempo is to imagine that you are walking at a fairly brisk pace. Each time you make a step, you would replicate this timing on the exercise movement that you are performing. A good gauge while looking at the timer is to complete a full rep every two seconds, one second to get to the top of movement and another to return to the start position.

This is the ideal tempo, and what we should aim for, but it's common with this type of exercise method for the trainer to fatigue, causing a loss of concentration on exercise form. When this happens, the tempo is maintained, but the exercise form suffers and full range of motion is lost, meaning we would be doing half reps and not working the muscle group to its full potential. In this situation, it's best to slow the tempo slightly in order to maintain form. This will help with muscle toning in a big way, whilst also maintaining our elevated heart rate for fat loss.

For the best possible start, take some time to become familiar with the exercises in any workout and practice each movement before you start. Here are the exercises listed on the program card:

Note: The following exercises are continuous movements that should maintain a steady tempo for a set amount of time. It's also important to maintain a steady, continuous breathing pattern.

Alternate toe tap

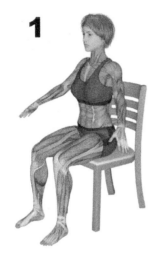

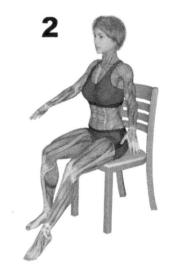

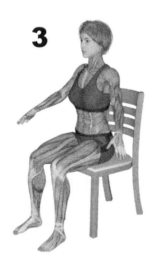

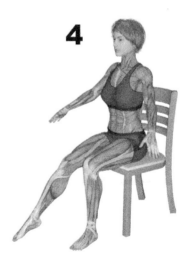

1 – Arms can be by your sides for balance or crossed across your chest. Maintain the default position

2 – Lift your right foot off the floor and straighten your leg by bending at the knee. Push your foot forward to tap the floor with your toes

3 – Return to the start position

4 - Lift your left foot off the floor and straighten your leg by bending at the knee. Push your foot forward to tap the floor with your toes

Scan code for animated image

Toe tap & flys

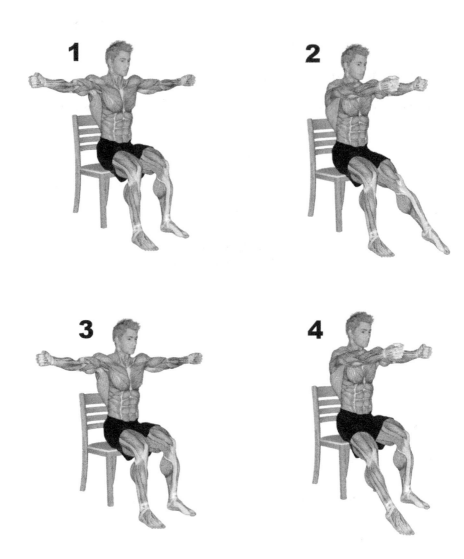

1 – From the default position, raise your arms so they are parallel to the floor and directly out to your sides. Make fists with your hands so your palms are facing forward

2 – Bring your fists together in front of your body (keeping your arms parallel to the floor). As you do this, lift your left foot off the floor and straighten your leg by bending at the knee. Push your foot forward to tap the floor with your toes

3 – Return to the start position

4 – Repeat step "2" but use your right foot to step forward

Scan code for animated image

Seated jacks

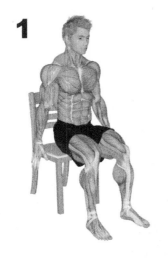

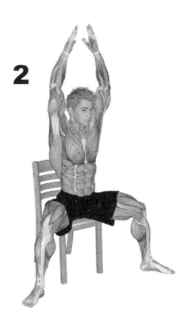

1 – Start in the default position with your arms by your sides, palms facing inwards

2 – As you exhale, lift both feet off the floor slightly and push your knees outwards, ensuring your lower legs stay below your quads. As you do this, bring your straight arms directly above your head from your sides, while twisting your palms to clap your hands at the top of the movement

3 – Return to the start position

Scan code for animated image

Toe tap, bicep curl

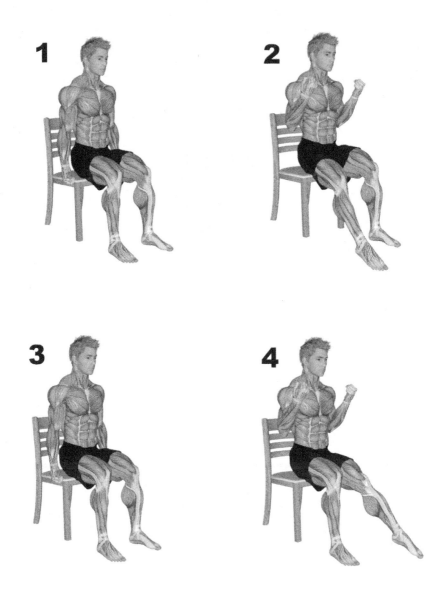

1 – From the default position, keep your arms by your sides, make fists with your hands and position your palms so they are facing forward

2 – As you exhale, bring your forearms up towards your upper arms. Your upper arms should stay fixed in the start position. While you do this, lift your right foot off the floor and straighten your leg by bending at the knee. Push your foot forward to tap the floor with your toes

3 – Return to the start position

4 – Repeat step "2" but use your left foot to step forward

Scan code for animated image

Toe tap, lateral raise

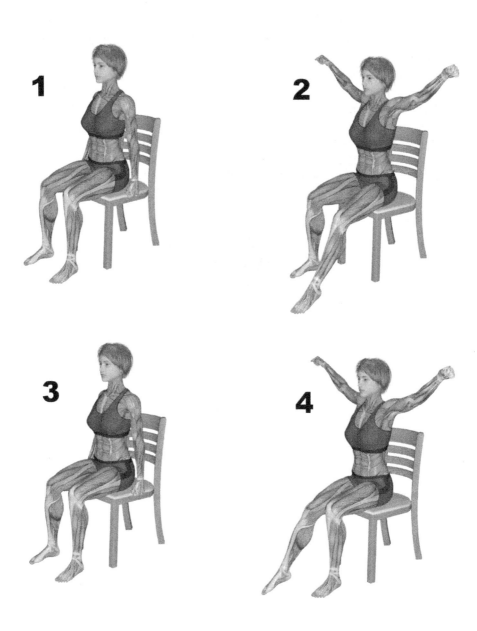

1 – From the default position, set your arms straight and by your sides. Make fists with your hands and have your palms facing inwards

2 – As you exhale, raise your arms out to your sides until your fists are just above head height. While you do this, lift your left foot off the floor and straighten your leg by bending at the knee. Push your foot forward to tap the floor with your toes

3 – Return to the start position

4 – Repeat step "2" but use your right foot to step forward

Scan code for animated image

Reach & pull

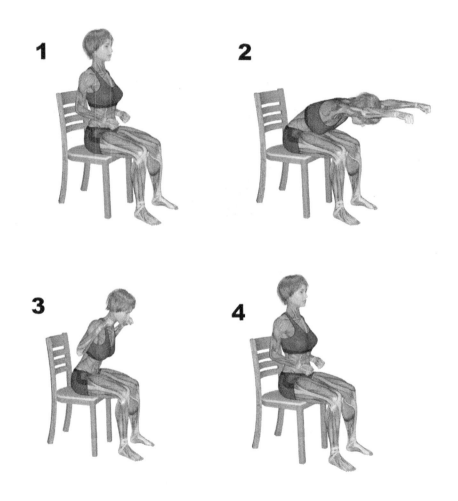

1 – From the default position, position your upper arms so they are by your sides, bend at the elbows so your lower arms are in front of you and parallel with the floor. Make fists with your hands, palms facing inwards

2 – As you exhale, hinge at the hips to move your upper body forward. While you do this, twist your shoulders to bring your upper arms to the side of your head

3 – Pull your fists towards your shoulders and pull your shoulders back and down. As you do this, hinge at the hips to bring your upper body closer to the start position

4 – Return to the start position

Scan code for animated image

Alternate elbow to knee

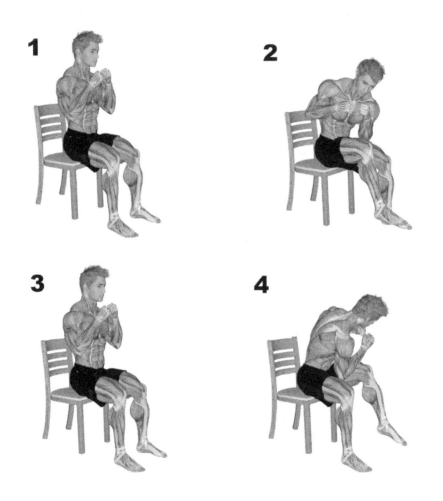

1 – From the default position, bring your lower arms towards your upper chest; make fists with your hands, palms facing inwards

2 – As you exhale, twist your upper body to your right, lower your upper body towards your right knee. While you do this, bring your right knee towards your left elbow by lifting your right leg

3 – Return to the start position as you inhale

4 – Exhale, twist your upper body to your left, lower your upper body towards your left knee. While you do this, bring your left knee towards your left elbow by lifting your left leg. Return to the start position as you inhale

Scan code for animated image

Double knee to chest

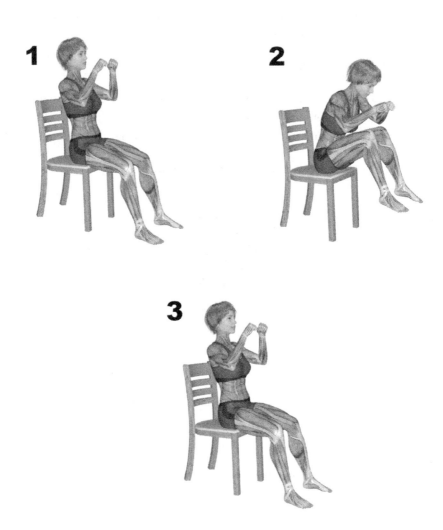

1 – From the default position, hinge at the hips to bring your upper body towards the back of the chair. You should feel the point of gravity through your glutes. Raise your feet off the floor slightly. You should feel an engagement of your abdominals

2 – As you exhale, lift both feet off the floor, bringing your knees towards your chest. As you do this, hinge at the hips to bring your upper body towards your knees

3 – Return to the start position as you inhale

Scan code for animated image

Exercise for Longevity and function

Exercise for function and longevity can technically be any type of exercise, but my definition of functional exercise is to develop movement and stability through every muscle group and joint. This is something that everyone will benefit from. Developing range of movement by performing exercises that challenge our bodies in the way they were designed to move will not only keep us supple, but a positive side effect will be the development of basic muscle strength.

So, looking back at the "workload & fitness goals" "workload & fitness goals", to align our training to fit this specific goal, we need to:

- Use timed exercises – 30 seconds to 1 minute per exercise
- Train partial or full body in each workout
- Workout length is subject to the individual
- Resistance can be added to some movements, but this is not essential

For this routine, we will work within a "sets and timeframe" range, rather than a "sets and reps" method and the exercises will prioritise range of movement and exercise form over everything else. Although we still aim to work inside a timeframe, this is variable depending on the individual. Yes, more time spent performing each exercise will challenge us more, but performing the exercises regularly and correctly is the most important thing here. Also, while working through these exercises, making a conscious effort to feel muscle groups working during exercise will increase our rate of progress greatly.

This is what the routine looks like:

LONGEVITY AND FUNCTION			

ROUTINE #			

MUSCLE GROUP	EXERCISE	SETS	TIME
CHEST, SHOULDERS	CHEST OPENING	3	30
MULTIPLE GROUPS	VOLCANO POSE	3	30
LEGS	CHAIR SQUATS	3	30
LOWER ABS	ALTERNATE LEG LIFT	3	30
MULTIPLE GROUPS	WARRIOR POSE	3	30
BACK, NECK	ROLL DOWN	3	30

WEEKS	MON	TUE	WED	THURS	FRI	SAT	SUN
1	*			*			
2	*			*			
3	*		*		*		
4	*	*	*		*	*	
5	*	*	*	*	*	*	*
6	*	*	*	*	*	*	*

How it works – In this routine, we will follow the exercise order starting with "chest opening" and finishing with "Roll down". We will be performing each exercise three times, for thirty seconds each (3 sets of 30 seconds). Once we have finished a thirty-second set, we can rest for ten – thirty seconds, then start another set of the same exercise, or move onto the next one if we have completed 3 sets.

Due to the nature of this exercise, most people can perform this workout every day. For total beginners, I would advise starting with a few days per week and working up to a daily pattern over time. This suggestion is reflected in the training schedule at the bottom of the workout card. Some trainers following this routine will see quick results and may want to progress faster, as they will soon outgrow the workload.

Tempo – When compared to the previous routine "weight loss and muscle tone", when performing exercise movements, the tempo doesn't have to be as continuous. When performing the exercises in this plan, we should move through the exercises slowly and with control. Once we reach the "top of movement" we hold for a second or two before slowly returning to the start position. It doesn't matter how many times we repeat the exercise (the amount of reps we do), it matters that we reach full range of movement through the exercise. The time is used as a guide only. If we are mid movement, when the time is up, we finish the exercise before resting. Adjusting the up or down time for exercises that we are stronger or weaker on, respectively, is a great tool for tracking progress.

This exercise routine is designed to engage major muscle groups and a wide range of stabiliser muscles while working to develop full body range of movement for stability, balance and general function.

Here are the exercises for this routine:

Chest opening

Start

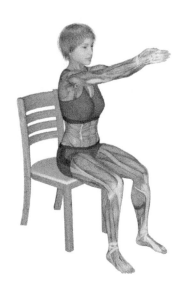

Top of movement

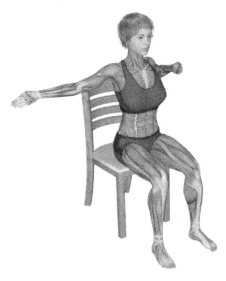

- From the default position, ensure your arms are straight and raise them out to your front so they are just above parallel with the floor
- Rotate your palms so they are facing inwards and in contact with each other
- Push your shoulders forward. This should push your palms further away from your upper body
- As you exhale, open your arms, bringing them past your sides and slightly down
- During this movement, you should feel your shoulders being pulled backwards, allow this to happen naturally
- Near the top of the movement, slowly push your shoulders back and down while pushing your chest forward
- Pause briefly at the top of movement before inhaling and returning to the start position

Scan code for animated image

Volcano pose

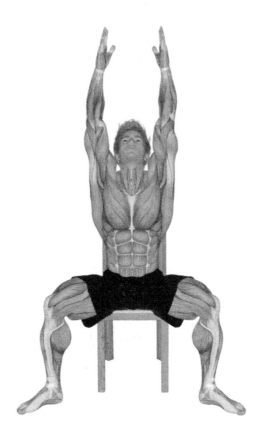

- From the default position, push your knees away from your mid line and plant your feet on the floor, toes facing outward. In this position, your upper and lower legs should still form a right angle and your lower legs should align with your upper legs
- Reach directly above your head with both arms, keeping them straight. Your palms should be turned inwards
- Once in this position, ensuring you keep a flat back, tilt your head backwards to look directly up
- Hold this position for your planned timeframe and keep your breathing controlled
- Once you have completed your set, slowly reverse the movement until you return to the start position

Chair squats

Start

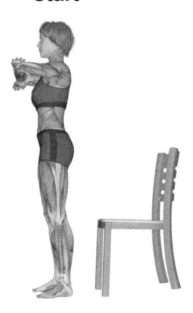

Top of movement

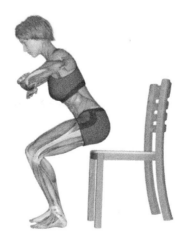

- Stand upright in front of the chair as if you were about to take a seat (The first stage of the default position)
- Cross your arms in front of you as per the illustration or raise your arms to your sides and slightly in front of you for balance
- Your feet should be about shoulder width apart and toes slightly turned outwards
- Keep your back flat, as you inhale, hinge at the hips slightly to push your glutes backwards bend at the knees to lower your glutes towards the chair
- Continue this lowering movement until your glutes "graze" the seat of the chair, but do not sit down. Hold your body weight with your quads
- Once at the top of movement, as you exhale, return to the start position

*** Note that if you are unable to make contact with the seat with your glutes, continue the movement to the point you are able, but try to make the full movement your goal. You can try to get a bit lower with each repetition or set.

Scan code for animated image

Alternate leg lift

Start

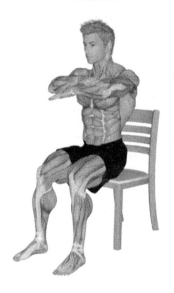

Top of movement

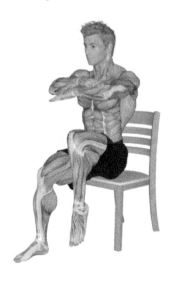

- From the default position, cross your arms in front of you so they are in line with your mid chest
- Lift your right foot away from the floor while maintaining the rest of your body positioning
- Continue to raise your knee towards your upper body while keeping your lower leg pointing directly downward. You may need to bend at the knee to do this
- Once you are close to the top of movement, bend at your ankle to point your toes down
- Pause at the top of movement before reversing the process and returning to the start position
- Once back at the start position, repeat on the left leg

Scan code for animated image

Warrior pose

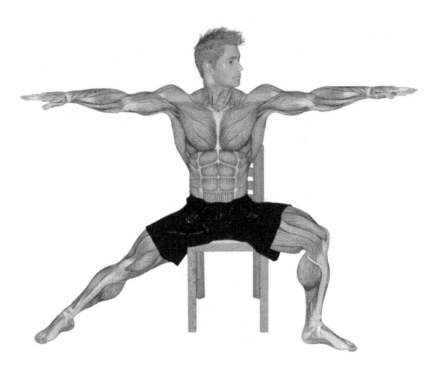

- From the default position, push your left knee towards your left side using movement from your hip. Plant your left foot on the floor. You should have a right angle between your upper and lower leg, toes should face the same direction as your left knee
- Straighten your right leg and rotate your hip to bring your right leg in line with your side. Twist your hip and rotate your ankle so your right foot is flat on the floor, toes slightly turned out, but facing the same direction as your knee
- Raise your upper arms so they are straight and directly out towards your sides. Your arms should be parallel with the floor, palms facing downwards
- Turn your head to look directly at your left hand

- Once you have built the position, hold for your planned timeframe, whilst maintaining a flat back and engaged core. Breathing should be controlled throughout the movement

Roll down

Start

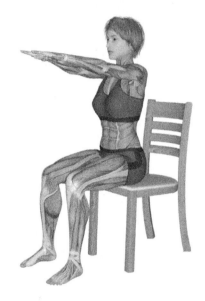

Top of movement

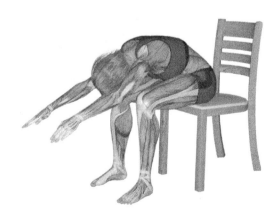

66

- From the default position, lift your straight arms out in front of you so they are just above parallel with the floor, palms facing downwards
- From this position, slowly bring your chin towards your upper chest by tilting your head forward
- Once you have a complete "chin tuck" start to round your back, pushing your shoulders towards your hips
- Continue the rounding of the back in sections from top to bottom until you reach your lower back
- You can choose to keep your arms above your head or lower them slightly during this movement
- Once at the top of movement, pause slightly while controlling your breathing before reversing the process and returning to the start position

*** Note that this exercise should be performed slowly and with control. Some people may find it more difficult to engage certain parts of the movement than others. A roll down starts with movement of the neck and continues in sections down the spine. Concentrating on rounding the spine a section at a time, from top to bottom, will help to develop this movement.

Scan code for animated image

Exercise for strength and muscle gain

A foundation of functional strength and muscle gain will be developed by performing any type of exercise in this exercise book. But if our fitness goal is to increase strength and size, we should explore the option of adding extra resistance to certain exercise movements.

Technically, strength and muscle gain are two different fitness goals. The reason I have linked them in this routine is because it's difficult to gain muscle without strength and the training involved for both strength and muscle gain goals uses the same method. It's worth mentioning that, generally speaking, the stronger we get, the more opportunity we have to build muscle, and muscle strength will always be the first training effect.

As per the information in the "Workload & fitness goals" chapter, we know that we should:

- Use "sets and reps" training method
- Train partial or full body workouts
- Workout length is subject to the individual
- Additional resistance should be used to overload the muscle

The "sets and reps" training method is important for this goal, as we want to overload each muscle group with resistance the best we can during our workouts. For each exercise, we would complete a set of 10 – 15 repetitions, have a short rest and repeat until we have completed 3 – 4 sets of the same exercise, before moving onto the next exercise.

We can train full body each session or we can train partial body. For this example, I will outline a "2-day split". This is where we will train four times per week, hitting each major muscle group twice per week. We will work from two separate routine cards, one marked "A" and the other marked "B".

Adding resistance is another very important part of strength and muscle gain goals. As mentioned in an earlier chapter, there are several ways to do this, but resistance bands are going to be our main choice. This is because with resistance bands, we have the option of anchor points. We can set the resistance band at an elevated level by attaching the door anchor (that is included in every good exercise band set) to the top, middle or bottom of a door, we can stand on the band or use other solid objects for anchor points. This gives us options and angles of resistance that are not available when using dumbbells or barbells, which opens up opportunities to a wider range of exercise choices.

With this said, if you are lucky enough to own a set of dumbbells, there are some exercise choices in this routine that can be performed with dumbbells or resistance bands, so you have extra options. This will be mentioned in the relevant exercise descriptions.

This is the routine card:

STRENGTH & MUSCLE GAIN			

ROUTINE #		

MUSCLE GROUP	EXERCISE	SETS	REPS
WORKOUT A			
CHEST	CHEST PRESS	3	10
CHEST	FLYS	3	10
BACK	LAT PULL DOWN	3	10
BACK	ROW	3	10
BICEPS	BICEP CURL	3	10
WORKOUT B			
TRICEPS	TRICEP PUSH DOWN	3	10
SHOULDERS	LATERAL RAISES	3	10
SHOULDERS	SHOULDER PRESS	3	10
LEGS	LEG EXTENSION	3	10
LEGS	CALF RAISES	3	10

WEEKS	MON	TUE	WED	THURS	FRI	SAT	SUN
1	A	B		A	B		
2	A	B		A	B		
3	A	B		A	B		
4	A	B		A	B		
5	A	B		A	B		
6	A	B		A	B		

How it works - Workout "A" is performed twice per week with several days in between this routine. Workout "A" targets the chest, back and bicep muscles. Workout "B" is also performed twice per week, with several days in between. Workout "B" targets the triceps, shoulders and legs. There are no set rules for creating a 2-day spilt, but it makes sense to split the muscle groups up the best you can by using synergists in the same workout. An example from this routine would be using back and bicep exercises in workout "A" as most compound back exercises also use the biceps in each rep.

For larger muscle groups, the exercise order is set so the same muscle group is targeted with consecutive exercises. This will increase intensity and overload on that group aligning the training with the goal.

The sets and reps are marked as "3 sets of 10 reps". This is a good start, but if you are following this routine, and you find this is not challenging enough, you can increase either the sets, reps, both. We should also be looking to increase the resistance level where possible. This is very subjective, so is not possible to give exact resistance as everyone is different, but, ideally, the resistance level we should be working at should see us near failure on the last few reps of each set. In this sense, failure means that we struggle to maintain our exercise form and range of movement because of the resistance level. This concept is another important factor when working towards strength and muscle gain fitness goals.

Training days - As we are training the same muscle group with multiple exercises, and multiple times per week, there are "rest" days between each "A / B" pattern. This gives us enough time to recover before going again.

Anchor points – As we are using resistance bands as the main form of resistance, these exercises call for an anchor point of some kind. With free weights, we generally work against gravity. This is always directly downwards, so we would move the weight, or resistance, away from the floor. Resistance bands give us the opportunity to create an opposing force from many angles, so we are less restricted. We do this by creating an anchor point.

Most good exercise band kits come with a door anchor. This is an attachment that we can attach to the top, middle, or bottom of a door to create a proxy point of gravity. Several exercises in the following routine have anchor points at the top and several have anchor points at the bottom of a door. The position of this point depends on the movement we are performing.

71

Some exercises will not need a door anchor, but they will need a fixed point. These movements use our feet to anchor the band. When standing on a band to create an anchor point, it's important that we have even lengths on either side of our feet so that we have equal resistance levels on both sides. It's also important for the longevity of a resistance band that we stand directly on and off it avoiding movement our feet from side to side whilst it is fixed as this can cause unnecessary wear on the band.

Here are the exercises for this workout routine:

Chest press

Start

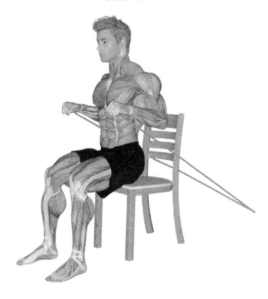

Top of movement

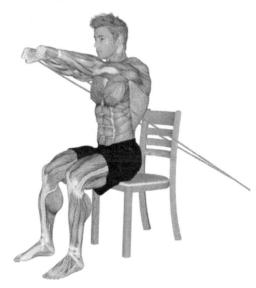

- Loop a resistance band through a door anchor. Attach the anchor to the bottom of a door
- Position the chair so the back is close to the door or anchor point, and at a distance that gives tension to the band from the start position
- Attach stirrups to the band or simply grip the ends
- From the default position, lift your lower arms so they are just above parallel with the floor, palms facing downwards
- Keep your upper arms by your sides. Keep your shoulders back and down
- As you exhale, push your fists out and slightly up in front of you, bringing them towards your midline until they make contact with each other at the top of movement
- At the top of movement, your arms should be straight, fists touching and positioned around head height
- Once at the top of movement, as you inhale, reverse the movement and return to the start position

Scan code for animated image

Flys

Start

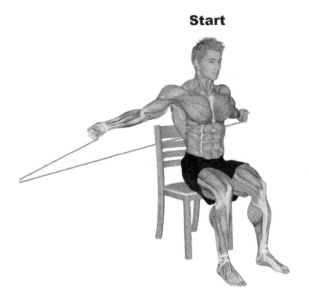

Top of movement

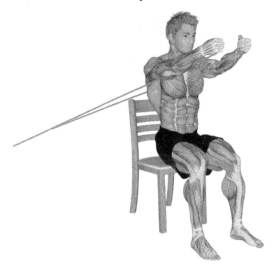

- Loop a resistance band through a door anchor. Attach the anchor to the bottom of a door
- Position the chair so the back is close to the door or anchor point, and at a distance that gives tension to the band from the start position
- Grip the ends of the band from the default position. Raise your straight arms out to your sides so they are just below parallel with the floor. Twist your palms so they are facing forward
- As you exhale, bring your straight arms towards your midline and slightly upwards
- You will reach the top of movement when your fists touch each other at about head height
- As you inhale, return to the start position

Scan code for animated image

Lat pull down

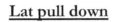

Start

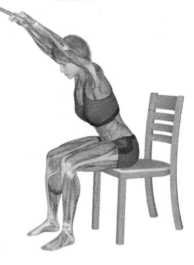

Top of movement

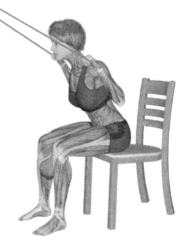

- Attach a door anchor to the top of a door and loop an exercise band through
- Position the chair so it is at enough distance to put tension on the band from the start position and grip the ends of the band
- From the default position, hinge at the hips slightly to move your upper body forward
- Lift your hands above your head with straight arms, balms facing forward
- As you exhale, pull your fists towards the sides of your shoulders. As you do this, push your chest forward slightly
- Once at the top of movement, as you inhale, return to the start position

Scan code for animated image

Row

Start

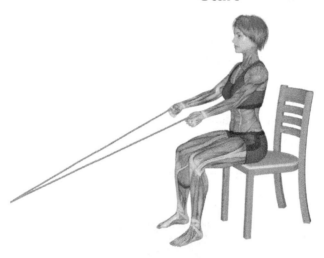

Top of movement

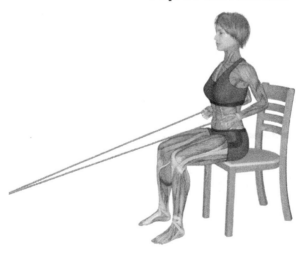

- Attach a door anchor to the bottom of a door and loop an exercise band through. Grip the ends of the band
- From the default position, move your arms forward so they are straight in front of you, at a slight angle towards the floor
- Your palms should be facing inwards and your arms should be about hip width apart
- As you exhale, pull your fists towards your navel. As you do this, push your shoulders back and chest forward slightly
- Once at the top of movement, inhale and return to the start position

Scan code for animated image

Bicep curl

Start

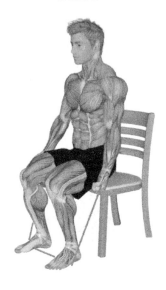

Top of movement

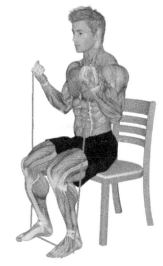

- This exercise also works well with dumbbells
- Select an exercise band and from the default position. Place the band under your feet to secure it in place
- There should be even lengths at either side of the band
- Grip the ends of the band so there is tension from the start position (You may need to wrap the band around your hands a few times to achieve this)
- Ensure your arms are almost straight by your sides, maintain a slight bend in the elbows, palms facing forward
- Push your shoulders back and down
- As you exhale, bring your lower arms up to meet your upper arms by bending at the elbows
- Maintain your upper arm and palm position. At the top of movement, your palms should face your shoulders
- Once at the top of movement, as you inhale, return to the start position

Scan code for animated image

Tricep pushdown

Start

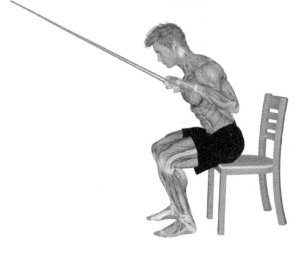

Top of movement

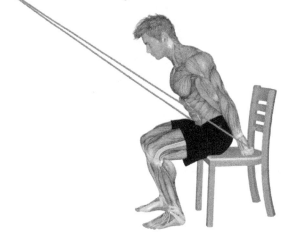

- Attach a door anchor to the top of a door and loop an exercise band through and grip the ends of the band
- From the default position, hinge forward at the hips slightly and raise your lower arms by bending at the elbows. Keep your upper arms by your sides, palms should face downwards
- From this position, pull your shoulders back and push your elbows back so they are slightly higher that your back
- As you exhale, straighten your arms, ensuring your upper arms maintain their position
- At the top of movement, your palms should be facing backwards
- Inhale and return to the start position

Scan code for animated image

Lateral raise

Start

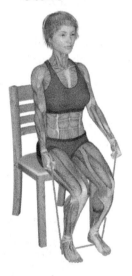

Top of movement

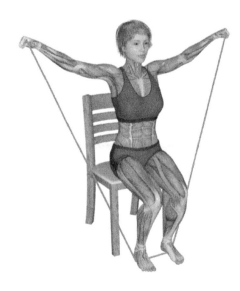

- This exercise also works well with dumbbells
- Select a resistance band. From the default position, plant your feet on the band to secure it in place. Ensure there are even lengths on either side of the band
- Grip the ends of the band. Position your arms so they are straight with a slight bend in the elbows and down by your sides and palms facing inwards
- As you exhale, raise your arms out towards your sides until they are just above parallel with the floor. You should keep a slight bend in the elbows and palms should be facing downwards at the top of movement
- Inhale and return to the start position after a slight pause at the top of movement

Scan code for animated image

Shoulder press

Start

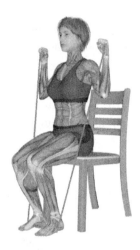

Top of movement

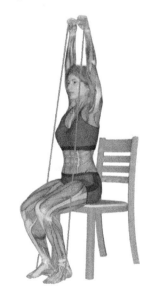

- This exercise also works well with dumbbells
- Select a resistance band and, from the default position, plant your feet on the band to secure it in place. Ensure there are even lengths on either side of the band
- Grip the ends of the band and raise your arms so your fists are in line with your chin, palms facing forward
- Your forearms should be pointing directly upwards and shoulders should be pushed back slightly
- As you exhale, push your fists directly above your head by straightening your arms
- Your fists should move towards each other naturally while performing this movement. They should touch each other at the top of movement
- Once at the top of movement, as you inhale, return to the start position

Scan code for animated image

Leg extension

Start

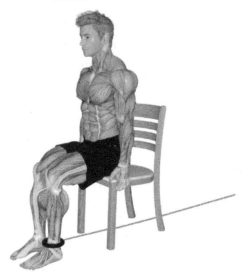

Top of movement

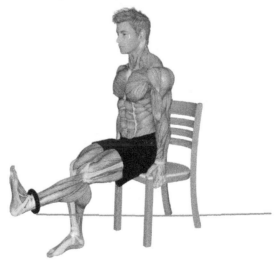

- Attach a door anchor to the bottom of a door, loop an exercise band through and attach an ankle strap to the opposite end
- Attach the ankle strap to the ankle of your working leg, ensuring the band runs underneath the chair
- From the default position, grip the sides of the chair for stability and lift your working leg off the floor slightly
- As you exhale, slowly straighten your working leg by bending at the knee. Ensure the quad of your working leg is parallel to the ground throughout the movement
- To increase the intensity of this exercise, pull your toes towards your shin at the top of movement
- Once at the top of movement, inhale and return to the start position
- Once you have completed a set, repeat on the opposite leg

Scan code for animated image

Calf raise

Start

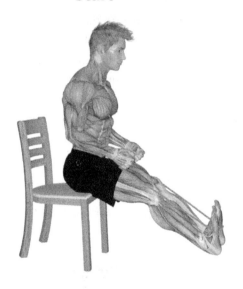

Top of movement

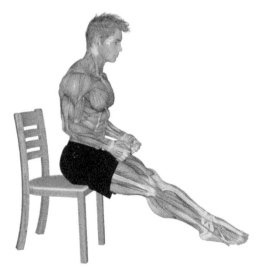

- From the default position, loop an exercise band around your feet. Ensure that you have even lengths of band on either side
- Straighten your legs so your heels are on the floor.
- Pull your toes towards your shins. At this point, make sure you have tension in the resistance band
- As you exhale, push your toes towards the floor by bending at the ankle
- At the top of movement, hold for a short pause before inhaling and returning to the start position

Scan code for animated image

Your personalised routine

Having a goal is important for all trainers. The routines in the previous chapters are based on specific goals with results in mind. These might be perfect for some trainers, but everyone's goal will be slightly different, so it's hard to create a "one size fits all" fitness routine.

If your goal is exactly as described in the example routines, and you feel the exercises and training schedule are a perfect fit, then, by all means, use this as your routine. But if your reasons for exploring chair workouts are broader or more niche, I'd encourage you to create your own routine from the theories and exercise choices in this book.

Maybe you would simply like to start any kind of chair exercise, but you are unsure of your specific fitness goals. In this case, I would suggest trying aspects of all the training types to see which you find the most enjoyable. There is nothing wrong with this; in fact, it's a great way to get started. After trying different types of training, most people will find something that they connect with and enjoy. It's also true to say that there may be aspects of training that some people will dislike. This is all part of the fitness journey, and any form of movement, provided it's performed with good form will be beneficial.

As previously mentioned, planning and prep is extremely important, so even if you are just dipping your toes into chair exercises, I would encourage you to try and pinpoint the exact reasons you want to engage in this form of training as a starting point, and then follow the advice that best fits your goals. I have also always been interested in hearing from readers of my guides. Helping people find a training direction, plan their routine and helping to solve problems when creating an exercise program is actually one of the highlights of this job for me. This is why I always welcome contact from anyone who reads my fitness guides. If you have an issue, or further questions, please give me a shout. I'm always happy to help where I can. You will find my contact information at the end of this book. ☺

If you would like to create your own workout routine, here are some blank exercise cards for personal use. They can be printed out, copied, or adjusted as you see fit. If you would like a PDF of these, I'm happy to send them to you.

ROUTINE #		

MUSCLE GROUP	EXERCISE	SETS	REPS

WEEKS	MON	TUE	WED	THURS	FRI	SAT	SUN
1							
2							
3							
4							
5							
6							

CIRCUIT TRAINING			

ROUTINE #			

MUSCLE GROUP	EXERCISE	REPS	SETS

WEEKS	MON	TUE	WED	THURS	FRI	SAT	SUN
1							
2							
3							
4							
5							
6							

2 DAY SPLIT			

ROUTINE #			

MUSCLE GROUP	EXERCISE	SETS	REPS
WORKOUT A			
WORKOUT B			

WEEKS	MON	TUE	WED	THURS	FRI	SAT	SUN
1							
2							
3							
4							
5							
6							

Progression

Whatever our fitness goals, as long as we consistently exercise with that goal in mind, we will progress. This progression will continue as long as we incrementally increase the challenge. If we stick to the same method of training, the same exercises and the same workload, we will reach what I like to call "maintenance mode", otherwise known as "a plateau".

For fitness goals such as function, balance, mobility and longevity, there is an element of progression in that, with the appropriate training, performed consistently over time, we will find it easier to reach a fuller range of movement, maintain a static hold for longer and our foundation muscle strength will increase. But, generally speaking, with this type of goal, we will eventually reach maintenance mode. For the purpose of this goal, as long as the exercise choices are right for us, they target our weakness or functions that we would like to improve, the same exercise routine can be performed indefinitely.

Some trainers training with this goal in mind will, however, want more progress. If you find yourself in this category, there are several things you can do:

- Increase the time on static holds
- Add more exercises to your routine
- Increase the sets per exercise
- Add an extra training day per week
- Explore other exercise techniques, such as strength training, etc.

For fitness goals such as strength building, muscle gain, and fat loss, we have to determine how strong, muscular, or lean we would like to become, respectively. Eventually, our original workout routine will not be enough of a challenge for further progress as we will have hit our "maintenance mode" or "plateau". Once we stop seeing increases in size, strength or fat loss, if we haven't reached our goals, we have to make changes to our training routines or diets for further progress.

If you find yourself in a position where you are no longer seeing progress with a strength and muscle gain goal, here are some ideas that can be used to break the plateau condition:

- Switch up exercise order by performing compound movements before isolation movements on each muscle group
- Increase resistance level
- Increase amount of sets per exercise
- Add exercises per muscle group into each workout
- Consider the use of free weights like dumbbells and barbells

Weight loss is always going to come down to "calories in vs calories out". In my experience, ninety percent of the result of weight loss or fat loss is determined in the kitchen. But an appropriate calorie intake coupled with more intense exercise can bring on excellent results, a lot quicker than diet alone.

Aside from an appropriate diet adjustment, to break a plateau on a weight loss goal, we could consider the following options:

- Increased time per exercise
- Increased sets of a circuit per workout
- Perform compound exercises (press and pull movements) at the start of a circuit
- More exercises per workout
- Increase workouts per week

In summary, whatever your level of commitment to exercise is, whether you want to go all in and achieve serious results, or whether you simply want to move more to become more active, having a pre-planned workout schedule in place will only ever help to serve you positively. If you only want to follow a few exercises, once per week, a completed exercise card will keep you on track and organised.

If you are committed to earning serious results through your training, these routine cards will not only keep you motivated, organised, accountable and focused, they can be upgraded as you develop, leaving the previous cards as a progress report.

More exercises

This section is dedicated to additional exercise choices that have not been included in the example workouts. You can use these in the creation of your own routine or switch out those in the example routines. Each exercise is listed under the main muscle group worked for easier navigation, and a separate section is reserved for yoga poses.

Where an exercise is illustrated with resistance bands, it's worth observing that the same movement can be performed without this equipment, so if you plan on using these movements, but do not want the extra resistance, simply ignore the reference to the bands. The movement will be the same.

Where dumbbells or free weights can be used, this is also mentioned in the description. Again, the exercise movement will be the same, so if you wish to use free weights, everything else in the description is relevant.

Back

Back extension

Start

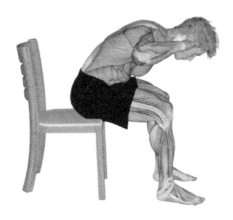

Top of movement

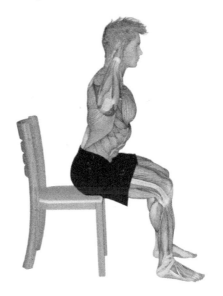

- From the default position, hinge forward from your hips to lower your upper body towards your knees
- Place your arms out to your sides and fingers on the sides of your head
- As you exhale, lift your upper body back towards the default position
- Once you reach the default position, slowly push your chest forward to arch your back
- Hold this position briefly before repeating the process

Scan code for animated image

High row

Start

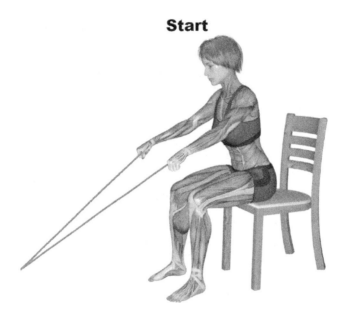

Top of movement

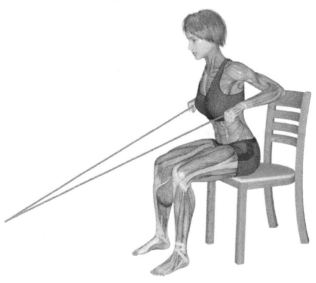

- Attach a door anchor to the bottom of a door and loop a resistance band through
- Facing the door, position your chair so there is tension in the band at the start position
- Grip the ends of the band with your palms facing downwards
- Hinge at the hips to position your upper body forward of the default position
- Straighten your arms in front of your upper body
- As you exhale, pull your fists in towards your mid chest, allowing your elbows to flare naturally to your sides
- Once at the top of movement, as you inhale, return to the start position

Scan code for animated image

Legs

Adduction/ abduction

Start

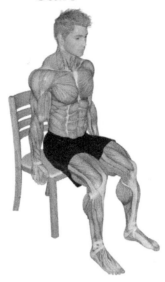

Top of movement

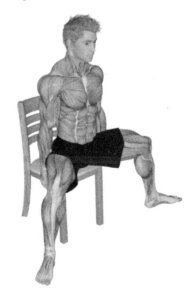

- Grip the sides of the chair for stability, hinge at the hips to bring your upper body slightly backwards from the default position. Your centre of gravity will shift through your glutes
- Lift both feet off the floor slightly so they are free to move without friction
- As you exhale, push your upper legs away from your midline
- Keep your knees above your feet as you perform this movement
- Once at the top of movement, as you inhale, return to the start position

Scan code for animated image

Leg curl

Start

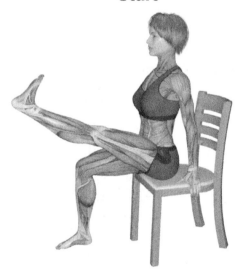

Top of movement

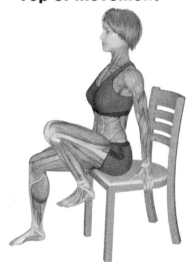

- From the default position, grip the sides of your chair for stability and lift your left leg off the floor
- With this leg raised, straighten it so it's out in front of you
- Pull the toes of your raised leg towards your shin to increase the intensity of this exercise
- As you exhale, bend your left leg at the knee to close the gap between your calf and your hamstring
- Your upper leg should remain in the start position throughout this exercise
- Once you are at the top of movement, as you inhale, return to the start position.
- On completion of your set, repeat on the other leg

Scan code for animated image

Leg press

Start

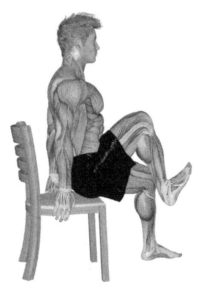

Top of movement

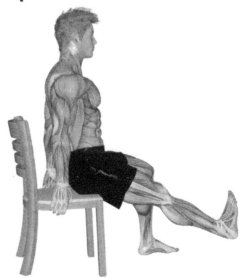

- From the default position, grip the sides of your chair for stability, hinge at the hips to position your upper body slightly backwards of the default position
- Lift your right leg off the floor to bring your knee closer to your upper body
- Pull the toes of your right leg towards your shin
- As you exhale, push your right leg forward and down to straighten it
- Continue this movement until the heel of your right leg makes a light contact with the floor
- Your toes should remain pointed towards your shin throughout the movement
- Once at the top of movement, inhale and return to the start position
- Once you have completed your set, repeat on the opposite leg

Scan code for animated image

Arms

Tricep stretch

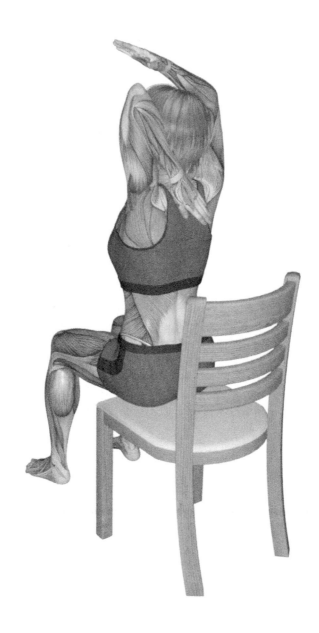

- From the default position, lift your left arm directly above your head, palm facing forward
- Bend your left arm at the elbow to place your palm behind your upper back
- Keep your upper left arm as close to vertical as you can
- To increase the stretch, some trainers will place their right hand on their left elbow and apply a small amount of pressure
- Hold this position for up to thirty seconds before repeating on the opposite arm

Overhead tricep extension

Start

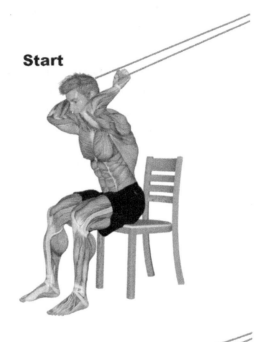

Top of movement

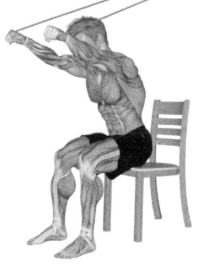

- Attach a door anchor to the top of a door and loop an exercise band through
- Position your chair back facing the door and ensure there is tension on the band at the start position
- From the default position, hinge slightly at the hips to position your upper body slightly forward of the default position
- Gripping the ends of the band, lift your arms up to your front to position the backs of your upper arms (triceps) so they are facing downwards and at about a forty-five degree angle from the floor
- At this point, your palms should be facing directly upwards as your arms should be bent at the elbows
- As you exhale, keep your upper arms fixed in the start position and straighten your arms through the elbows
- At the top of movement, your upper arms should still be in the start position and your palms should be facing the floor
- As you inhale, return to the start position

Scan code for animated image

Drag curl

Start

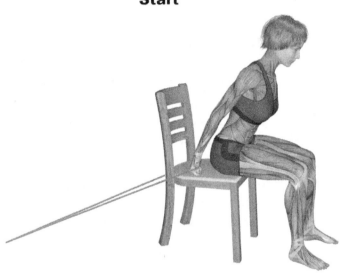

Top of movement

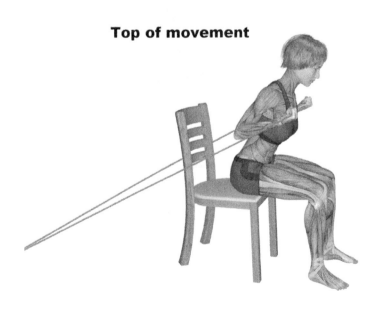

122

- This exercise can be performed with dumbbells or hand weights
- Attach a door anchor to the bottom of a door, loop an exercise band through and position your chair so the back is facing the door
- From the default position, hinge forward slightly at the hips
- Pull your shoulders back and rotate your shoulders to place your arms slightly to your rear
- Straighten your arms at the elbows and ensure your palms are facing forward
- As you exhale, maintain your upper arm position and bend at your elbows to bring your fists towards your shoulders
- At the top of movement, your palms should face your shoulders and upper arms should have maintained their position
- As you inhale, return to the start position

Scan code for animated image

Tricep dips

Start

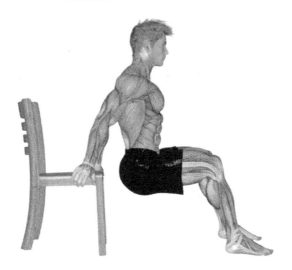

Top of movement

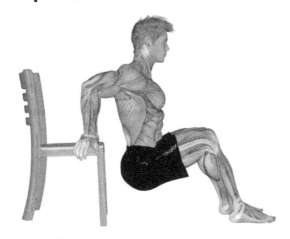

** This is an advanced exercise that requires a good foundation of upper body strength.

- Position your chair against a wall for extra stability
- Starting with the chair to your rear, grip the sides of the chair to take your body weight through your arms
- Your feet should be firmly planted on the floor, about shoulder width apart
- Your legs should be bent at the knees at, or just past a right angle
- This will leave your upper body suspended just in front of the chair
- As you inhale, lower your upper body and glutes towards the ground by bending at the elbows
- Allow your elbows to flare out to your sides naturally.
- There will be some movement through your shoulders, but you should not continue to lower if you feel pain in this area
- Keep your feet planted firmly on the ground throughout the exercise
- Once you are at the top of movement, exhale and return to the start position

Scan code for animated image

Shoulders

Upright row

Start

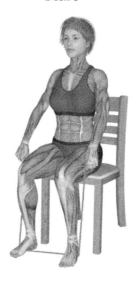

Top of movement

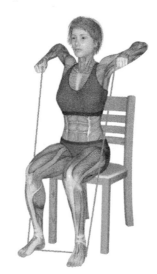

- This exercise can be performed with dumbbells
- From the default position, bring your feet slightly closer to the chair and secure a resistance band underneath them, ensuring there are equal lengths on either side. Plant your feet firmly on the floor
- Grip the ends of the band so your arms are straight and run to the side of your body towards the anchor point of the band
- Your palms should face backwards
- As you exhale, pull the band up and backwards, bending at your elbows and lifting your shoulders
- Allow your elbows to flare out to your sides
- Once at the top of movement, inhale and return to the start position

Scan code for animated image

Front raise

Start

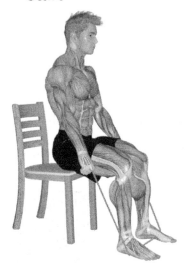

Top of movement

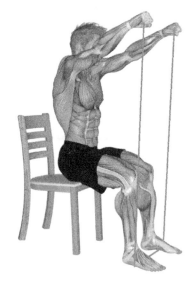

- This exercise can be performed with dumbbells or other free weights
- From the default position, secure an exercise band beneath your feet, planting your feet firmly on the ground
- Grip the ends of the band with straight arms by your sides and in line with the anchor point at your feet
- Your palms should be facing to your rear
- As you exhale, lift your arms in front of you until your fists are just above head height
- At the top of movement, your arms should be straight, with a slight bend in the elbows, and your palms should be facing downwards
- Once at the top of movement, as you inhale, return to the start position

Scan code for animated image

Reverse fly

Start

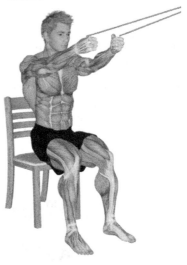

Top of movement

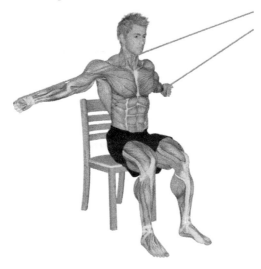

- Attach a door anchor to the top of a door and loop a resistance band through
- Face the door and grip the ends of the band, ensuring there is tension in the band from the start position
- Straighten your arms out in front of you so your palms are facing inwards. Your fists should be about head height and towards your midline
- As you exhale, while keeping your arms straight (with a slight bend in the elbows), pull your fists towards your sides, backwards and slightly down
- As you do this, push your chest forward for extra range of movement
- Once at the top of movement, inhale and return to the start position

Scan code for animated image

Abdominals

Seated crunch

Start

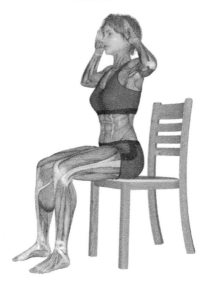

Top of movement

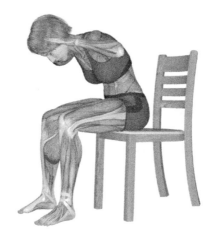

136

- From the default position, raise your arms so your fingers are resting on the sides of your head
- As you exhale, bring your upper body towards your upper legs by bending through your mid back
- Continue the movement until you slightly hinge at the hips
- Once at the top of movement, inhale as you return to the start position

Scan code for animated image

Waist twist

Start

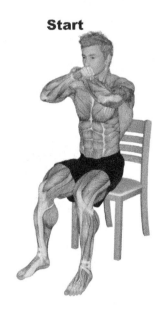

Top of movement

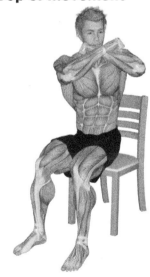

- From the default position, lift your arms and either cross them over your chest or place your fingers on the sides of your head
- As you exhale, keep your abdominals engaged and twist your upper body and shoulders to your left side
- Continue to build on the movement by following this twist through the lower section of your upper body
- You should keep your upper body vertically aligned as per the start position throughout the movement
- Once you have reached the top of movement, inhale and return to the start position
- Continue your set until you have completed your planned reps before repeating on the opposite side

Scan code for animated image

Side bend

Start

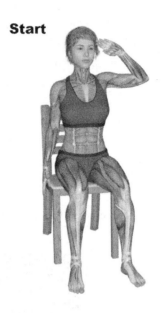

top of movement

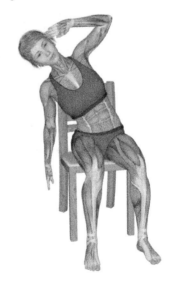

- From the default position, lift your left hand to place your fingertips on the left side of your head. Ensure that your bent arm is aligned directly to your side. This will help to keep your upper body from moving forward or backward during the exercise

- Your right arm should be straight and directly down by your right side

- As you exhale, lean your upper body towards your right-hand side by dropping your right shoulder downwards

- Continue the movement by lifting your right hip up slightly. You should feel the oblique's on your right-hand side contract and a stretch through your left-hand side

- Ensure that you maintain a neutral position in the sagittal plane (front and back movement)

- Finally, to finish the movement, and for an extra stretch on your left side, slowly tilt your head to the right

- Once you have reached the top of movement, inhale and return to the start position

- Once you have completed your set on this side, repeat in the opposite direction

Scan code for animated image

Yoga poses

Although the focus of this book is not on the practice of yoga, this exercise type fits nicely with chair workouts. I also believe that everyone can benefit from the functional movements and static holds that are an integral part of yoga.

It's for this reason that I have added several yoga poses for you to try out, or include in your own routine.

I will reiterate that the illustrated poses and descriptions in this guide are included with static holds in mind. This means that we would build a pose and hold it for a set period. It is possible, however, to build a pose and add small, controlled movements to a yoga exercise choice. Once a pose is built to our individual range of motion, we can move some or all of our working muscle groups with control further into the position, or back towards the start position.

For example, if we were to perform a warrior pose, and our current range of movement through our chest and shoulders does not allow us to place our arms directly out to our sides, we could build the position to our ability and while holding for our allotted time, slowly and with control, push our arms back to try to increase the range of movement.

This is an option that I would not advise for the total beginner. It may take some time to become familiar enough with the exercise and the body's ability before pushing for progress.

"Building the pose" is a phrase I like to use for this type of exercise. When performing a static hold that incorporates many muscle groups and planes of movement, there is much more value in working on a section at a time, rather than simply "getting into the pose". This is because we can give our full attention to each muscle group involved in the exercise, so there is less chance we will neglect certain areas. It also takes a lot of concentration to perform these exercises, and if we are conscious of our position, we will be more likely to address it during the timed hold if we fatigue in that area.

During a static hold yoga pose, maintain a steady breathing rhythm and think about how you built the pose; Are your feet and knees still aligned? Is your back set as per the start position? Etc. This only adds value to the exercise, as it makes us aware of our weaknesses and gives us the opportunity to address any issues right away. The more this is performed, the more proficient you will become at the exercise and the more natural it will feel, to the point that you will sense yourself losing alignment before it has happened.

The poses in this section are variations from commonly named yoga poses that focus on valuable movements not commonly used in everyday life, so most people will benefit from them.

Remember that if you would like to develop a certain pose but struggle when you start to use it, build the pose at your maximum range of motion and hold in this position for your planned timeframe. It will become more comfortable over time and you will be able to push further the more you practice. Partial poses are also an option. You can use sections of a pose if you are unable to perform the full pose. For example, if you see an exercise that uses full body engagement but are unable to perform the lower body section, placing your lower body in the default position and performing the upper body section is perfectly acceptable.

Pigeon pose

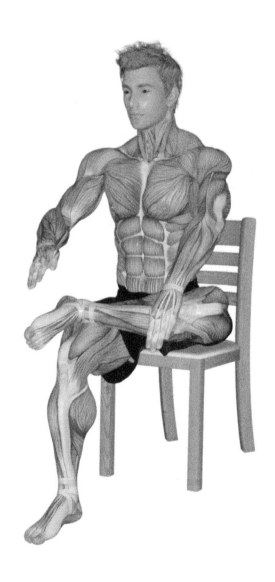

- From the default position, bring your left leg off the floor and bend at the knee
- Keep your right foot planted firmly on the floor
- Twist your hip to rest the outside of your left ankle just above your right knee
- Keep your back flat and upper body aligned as per the default position
- Use your right hand to hold your left ankle in place if you need to
- (Optional) Apply a small amount of pressure to your left knee to increase the range of movement
- Hold for your planned time before slowly reversing the movement back to the default position before repeating on the opposite leg

If the knee of your working leg points up at an angle, this is very common and not a problem. Hold the position only to the point that you are comfortable with. You can work towards lowering the knee over time.

Seated tree

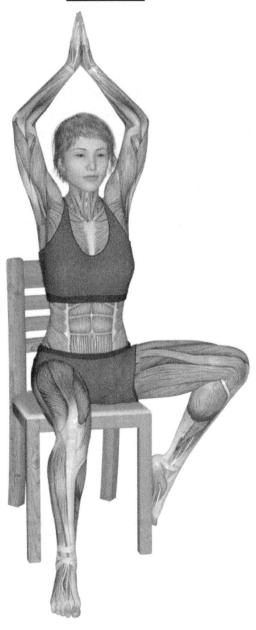

- From the default position, lift your left leg away from the floor by bending at the knee
- Rotate your left hip and bend your left ankle to place the sole of your left foot on the side of the left chair leg
- Ensure that your hips and torso remain forward, facing
- Keep your right foot planted firmly on the floor
- Engage your abdominals and core
- Raise both arms directly above your head
- Turn your palms inwards and place them together, fingers pointing directly up
- Hold for your planned time before returning to the default position
- Rebuild the pose with the opposite leg and repeat the build of your upper body to ensure both hips benefit from the same intensity

Half moon

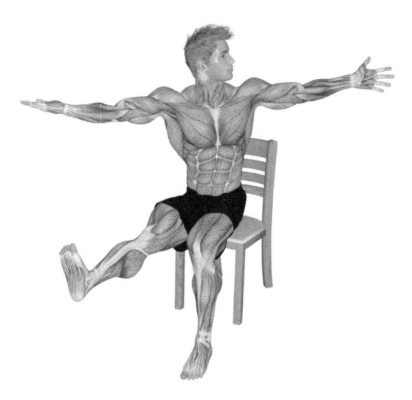

- From the default position, straighten your right leg by bending at the knee
- Keep your hips facing forward and abdominals and core engaged
- Raise both arms out to your sides so they are parallel with the floor
- Twist your right wrist so your palm is facing upwards
- Twist your left wrist so your palm is facing forward
- From this position, twist your torso to the left
- Once your torso twist has reached its maximum range of motion, turn your head to look directly down your left arm

- Hold this position for your planned time before returning to the default position and rebuilding with the opposite leg and twisting in the opposite direction

A couple of things to be aware of on this one: Make sure your straight leg doesn't drop. Be aware of your arm positioning; it's common to lose focus on your "palm up" arm as this is behind your head, it can drift forward or drop. Finally, be aware of your back and hip positioning when building the position and when holding; it's easy to round the back and rotate the hips, especially during the torso twist.

Camel

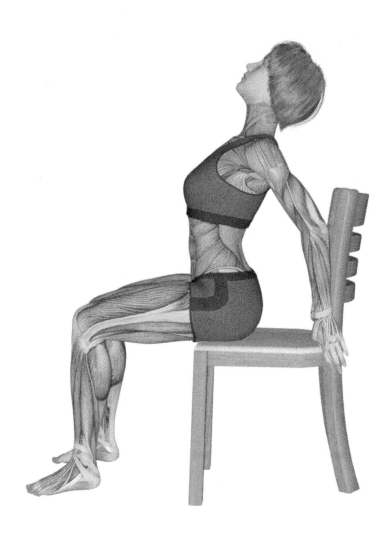

- Set up the default position so that your glutes are slightly further forward on the chair than normal. You will need the extra space behind you
- While maintaining your back alignment, push your arms backwards so you are able to grip the rear of the seat or the backrest of the chair
- Your palms should be facing inwards and arms straight or with a slight bend at the elbows
- As you exhale, push your chest up and forwards
- Continue this movement by pulling your shoulders back and down
- Once you have reached the limit of your range of motion in this movement, hold the position
- Once this position is stable, tilt your head to look upwards

Forward fold & prayer

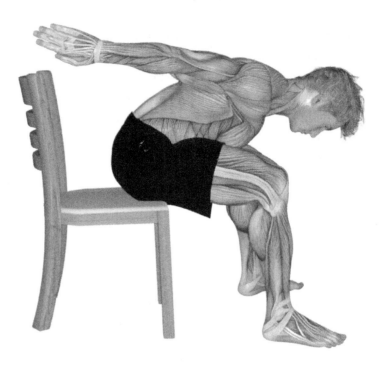

- Set up in the default position as usual, but position your feet on the floor slightly wider than hip width apart
- As you exhale, hinge at the hips to bring your upper body towards your upper legs
- Ensure you do not round the rest of your back when moving into this position and keep your head and neck in a neutral position
- Once you have reached your maximum range of movement with the forward fold, with straight arms, rotate your shoulders to bring your arms back and behind your torso, palms facing inwards
- At this point, you can either rest your fingertips on the backrest or pull your shoulders closer together to clasp the fingers of both hands together
- Hold this position for your planned timeframe and slowly reverse the process to return to the default position

This pose is great developing strength and mobility in the shoulders, lower back and core. As we can't see our arm position, it's common to let them bend more than we would like at the elbows, so this is something to be aware of. Also, this is a fairly tricky pose for a lot of people with lower back and shoulder issues, so the range of movement may differ fairly drastically from the diagram for some. Time and consistency with the exercise will always help.

Twist & prayer

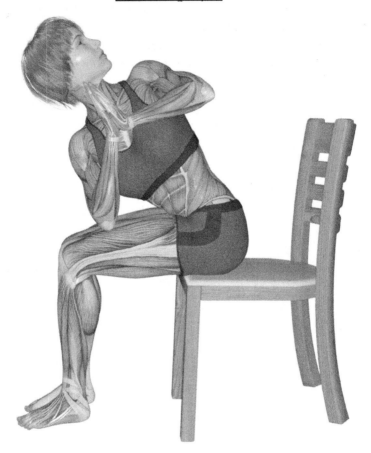

- Set up in the default position, but plant your feet on the floor close together. The insides of your feet, knees and upper legs should be touching each other
- From this position, twist at your waist towards your left-hand side until you reach your maximum range of movement
- Bring your palms into a prayer position (palms touching, fingers pointed upwards) close to your body and in line with your upper chest
- Turn your head to look at your left shoulder
- You can choose to hold the position at this point

- To develop the movement further, bend at the waist to drop your right elbow towards your left knee
- To increase shoulder mobility from here, shift your palms towards your left shoulder by pushing your right shoulder forward and left shoulder backwards
- Once you have held your chosen variation of this position, slowly return to the default position and repeat on the other side

Would you like to help me out?

I would like to take this opportunity to thank you for your interest in this guide. It means a great deal to me that you made the purchase. I hope that it has been useful and remember, I'm more than happy to help out further if you have questions about the training.

I'm a self-published fitness author, so have no backing from big publishing houses or investors. Each guide I create is my own work and is published using my own finances. Competition is fierce in this game, but you can help me out if you would like to?

Garnering online book reviews is extremely important for any author/ publisher in this day and age, so this is where I humbly ask you for some help. If you enjoyed this book and would like to support me, it would mean the world to me if you went back to the online bookstore where you picked up the guide to leave a star rating and a short review. A sentence or two about why you enjoyed the book or found it helpful would be more than enough.

This would help me out more than you know, and I would be eternally grateful.

Thanks again, you are the greatest! All the best.

Jim (James Atkinson)

Jim@jimshealthandmuscle.com

Something else you may be interested in?

If you would like to learn more about this series and my other books, you can do so by visiting my author page. Visit Amazon and search "James Atkinson". You will see my ugly mug, click it, and you will be taken to my page. Alternatively, just follow the link below - ☺

James Atkinson Author Page

You can stay up to date with my current activities, be alerted to deeply discounted, or free new release by signing up to my email list. When you sign up, there are a couple of short PDF guides related to diet and exercise that you may find useful. These get delivered as part of the sign-up process.

As we all know, diet plays a big part in health and fitness, and the two subjects fit hand in hand. So I would like to offer you a free download of seven healthy recipes that I created and use regularly myself. You can copy the recipes exactly, add your own twist to them, or simply take inspiration from them.

If you would like to grab this and become a part of my email list, you can do so by following the link below.

Take me to the 7 Healthy Recipes!

Don't worry, I never spam, and newsletters are infrequent, but there is always something of value inside when they do get sent.

Also by James Atkinson

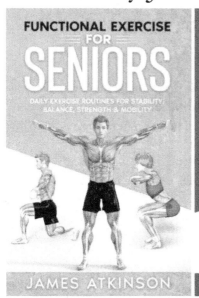

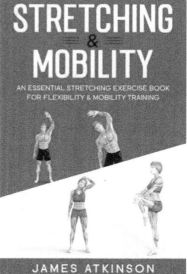

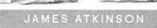

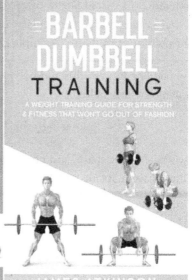

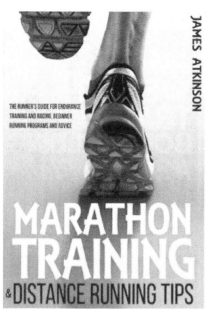

THE RUNNER'S GUIDE FOR ENDURANCE TRAINING AND RACING, BEGINNER RUNNING PROGRAMS AND ADVICE

JAMES ATKINSON

MARATHON TRAINING & DISTANCE RUNNING TIPS

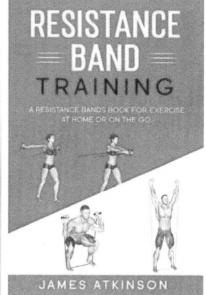

RESISTANCE BAND TRAINING

A RESISTANCE BANDS BOOK FOR EXERCISE AT HOME OR ON THE GO.

JAMES ATKINSON

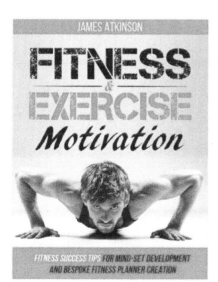

JAMES ATKINSON

FITNESS & EXERCISE Motivation

FITNESS SUCCESS TIPS FOR MIND-SET DEVELOPMENT AND BESPOKE FITNESS PLANNER CREATION

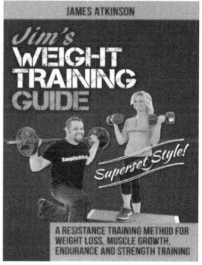

JAMES ATKINSON

Jim's WEIGHT TRAINING GUIDE

Superset Style!

A RESISTANCE TRAINING METHOD FOR WEIGHT LOSS, MUSCLE GROWTH, ENDURANCE AND STRENGTH TRAINING

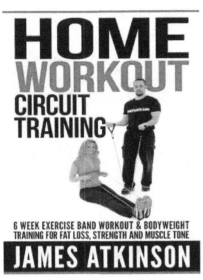

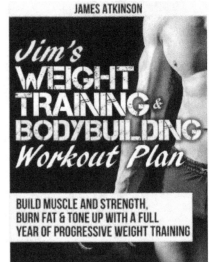

There is enough information in this fitness book to absorb and implement, but I want you to get results and I'm here to help you get to where you want to be in fitness! If you are not where you want to be and can't see a path, I have a free podcast where I chat about common issues and give advice on how to overcome and progress. I'd love to squeeze all the advice for everyone into a single guide, but this can detract from a goal and causing overwhelm. I've seen it many times and been there myself. Too many ideas can cause paralysis, causing no action to be taken at all.

If podcasts are your thing, I have one that addresses common issues with fitness progression. Each episode is read by myself highlighting a specific topic, giving actionable advice based on experience. Episode length is around twenty minutes. So let's chat! Get a coffee on, drop by and have a listen at:

AudioFitTest.com

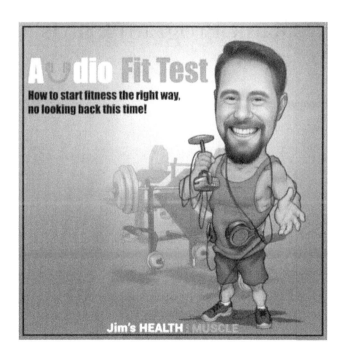

Blank Program Cards

ROUTINE #		

MUSCLE GROUP	EXERCISE	SETS	REPS

WEEKS	MON	TUE	WED	THURS	FRI	SAT	SUN
1							
2							
3							
4							
5							
6							

ROUTINE #	

MUSCLE GROUP	EXERCISE	SETS	REPS

WEEKS	MON	TUE	WED	THURS	FRI	SAT	SUN
1							
2							
3							
4							
5							
6							

CIRCUIT TRAINING

ROUTINE #		

MUSCLE GROUP	EXERCISE	REPS	SETS

WEEKS	MON	TUE	WED	THURS	FRI	SAT	SUN
1							
2							
3							
4							
5							
6							

CIRCUIT TRAINING			

ROUTINE #		

MUSCLE GROUP	EXERCISE	REPS	SETS

WEEKS	MON	TUE	WED	THURS	FRI	SAT	SUN
1							
2							
3							
4							
5							
6							

166

2 DAY SPLIT			

ROUTINE #			

MUSCLE GROUP	EXERCISE	SETS	REPS
WORKOUT A			
WORKOUT B			

WEEKS	MON	TUE	WED	THURS	FRI	SAT	SUN
1							
2							
3							
4							
5							
6							

167

2 DAY SPLIT			

ROUTINE #		

MUSCLE GROUP	EXERCISE	SETS	REPS
WORKOUT A			
WORKOUT B			

WEEKS	MON	TUE	WED	THURS	FRI	SAT	SUN
1							
2							
3							
4							
5							
6							

168

JIMSHEALTHANDMUSCLE.COM

PAPERBACK EDITION

ISBN: 978-0-9932791-9-5

PUBLISHED BY: JBA Publishing

http://www.JimsHealthAndMuscle.com

jim@jimshealthandmuscle.com

Chair workouts for every fitness level

First published in 2024

Made in the USA
Coppell, TX
04 November 2024

39618533R00098